ALSO BY BETTE HAGMAN

More from the Gluten-free Gourmet

The Gluten-free Gourmet Cooks Fast and Healthy

The Gluten-free Gourmet Bakes Bread

The Gluten-free Gourmet

BETTE HAGMAN

The Gluten-free Gourmet

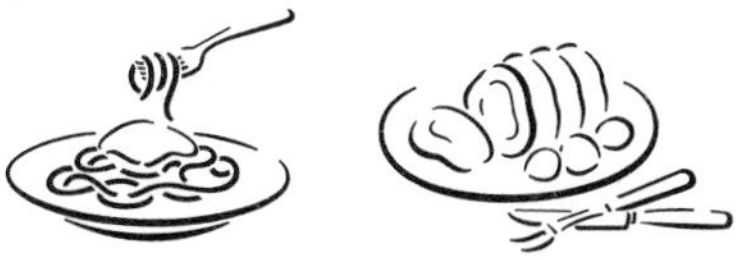

Living Well Without Wheat

REVISED EDITION

An Owl Book
Henry Holt New York

Henry Holt and Company, LLC
Publishers since 1866
115 West 18th Street
New York, New York 10011

Henry Holt® is a registered trademark
of Henry Holt and Company, LLC.

Distributed in Canada by H. B. Fenn and Company Ltd.

Library of Congress Cataloging-in-Publication Data
Hagman, Bette.
The gluten-free gourmet : living well without wheat /
by Bette Hagman.—Rev. ed.
p. cm.
Includes bibliographical references.
ISBN 0-8050-6484-2 (An Owl Book : pbk.)
1. Gluten-free diet—Recipes. I. Title.
RM237.9.H34 1990 89-20116
641.5'63—dc20 CIP

Henry Holt books are available for special promotions
and premiums. For details contact: Director, Special Markets.

First published in hardcover in 1990 by
Henry Holt and Company

Printed in the United States of America

3 5 7 9 10 8 6 4

The original Gluten-free Gourmet *was dedicated to my husband, Joe, who tactfully refrained from comment after tasting my first attempts at gluten-free baking, and to Donna Jo, a tester, who not only convinced me to "write a book" but taught me to cook.*

This revised edition is dedicated to a group of fellow celiacs who shared their time, their ideas, and their favorite recipes to make the revision a complete guide to Living Well Without Wheat.

Grateful thanks to

the Rochester Gang and Mary Lou

Contents

Foreword

"If the patient can be cured at all, it must be by means of diet." Not a surprising statement when it is recognized that dietary management was the primary and often sole treatment of gastrointestinal disorders 110 years ago; however, the author, Samuel Gee, an English physician, also specified that "the allowance of farinaceous [starchy] foods must be small." His treatise "On the Coeliac Affection," published in 1888, described and discussed sprue in such an incisive, accurate manner that the article became a classic example of medical writing. Unfortunately, another century passed before clinical observation and application of the developing scientific method eventually produced the answer to the myriad ills of celiac disease, idiopathic steatorrhea, nontropical sprue, adult celiac disease, gluten-induced enteropathy, all of which are now regarded as synonymous with celiac sprue.

Fifty years ago celiac disease was known only as a childhood disease characterized by symptoms of weight loss, malnutrition, and complaints of a voluminous, foul diarrhea. Those of us in medical school in the 1940s and early '50s remember it as one that was not readily understood but, for some unknown reason, was treated with a diet consisting mainly of bananas. It was hard to foresee that within the next few years its treatment would radically change, the intestinal pathology would be described, and its specific cause would be identified. Since celiac disease was a rarity in the United States, it did not create great interest, so Europe, where it was a more common problem, became the point of investigation from which came the knowledge regarding the diet and pathology leading to advancements in diagnosis and treatment.

The anatomical changes that typified celiac disease were first described on tissue samples from the small intestine obtained surgically, but within a few years simpler techniques for obtaining biopsies without an abdominal operation provided easier access to the upper small intestine. Knowledge of the specific pathological findings not only became evidence that classic childhood disease and adult celiac disease, previously classified as idiopathic steatorrhea, were the same, but also labeled the disease as "gluten-induced enteropathy," used synonymously with the term celiac disease. Because other, less common intestinal disorders can mimic these changes, the abnormalities found in the small bowel biopsy are not always absolutely specific for celiac disease, but when combined with a response to the gluten-free diet and/or a positive reaction to the serological tests available today, biopsy has become the "gold standard" for diagnosis. Different criteria for the diagnosis have evolved over the years, ranging from only a simple response to a gluten-free diet to the need for both an abnormal biopsy and a response to the diet. Other pediatricians earlier required an abnormal biopsy, a clinical response to the gluten-free diet, and then a repeat biopsy after two years to show a return to normal. Some physicians even felt that gluten should be reintroduced (gluten challenge) to be followed by recurrence of both the symptomatic state and the pathological findings. Today, the presence of the typical celiac pathology and a clinical response to the diet are unequivocal proof of the disease.

Celiac disease may be present without diarrhea, but it may announce itself as a symptom of the vitamin and/or mineral deficiencies that result from malabsorption. The most common of these are anemia, due to decreased iron or folic acid uptake, bone disease from a lack of calcium and/or vitamin D, or bleeding disorders resulting from the malabsorption of vitamin K. Such a typical presentation has been recognized and reported by certain investigators as "the many faces of sprue" or considered by others as "the great imitator." There is a more subtle association in patients with other diseases; that is, dermatitis herpetiformis, insulin-dependent diabetes mellitus, hypothyroidism, growth retardation, infertility in both men and women, multiple spontaneous abortions and increased stillbirths, and even in the presence of dental enamel defects, alopecia, and oral ulcerations. These deficiency manifestations and associations have become more common than those seen with the gastrointestinal and nutritional diseases, and therefore diagnosis largely depends on the attending physician's high index of suspicion. There is no doubt of a genetic connection because the presence of celiac disease in the relatives of those known to have the disease is definitely greater than in the general population. It also must not be forgotten that celiac disease can occur in those who are sixty years of age or older and that certain other autoimmune diseases often coexist with celiac disease.

Early studies in Europe reported a difference in the prevalence of celiac disease in different countries. With the development of specific antibodies and their use in mass screening, various populations have demonstrated less, if any, variability between countries and an increase in the numbers of asymptomatic, previously undiagnosed individuals. In Italy this technique revealed a ratio of known to unknown cases that was only one in seven, making it one of the most common chronic disorders in that country and coining the term "the celiac iceberg." The presence of this large number of heretofore unknown patients would explain the previous discrepancies not only in Europe but also in the United States. Unfortunately, mass screening in the United States has not been reported, but it has now been accepted internationally that determining the prevalence of celiac disease should be based on serological testing to identify those with the disorder to be confirmed later by a small bowel biopsy.

Recently new concepts have broadened the approach to celiac disease. Gluten sensitivity is considered active whether the symptoms are full blown or at the absolute minimum. Silent celiacs are those without any discernible evidence of disease activity although they both have abnormal biopsies; however, a blending of new and old medical findings and new technological advances have led to anatomical observations in the pathology that run the gamut from the classical changes to what most pathologists would call normal. Even without the flattened villi the presence of a large number of lymphocytes within the mucosal cells differentiate this from an otherwise normal-appearing biopsy. These individuals, who were not all asymptomatic, had a history of active disease and an abnormal biopsy before recovering on a gluten-free diet with a normal biopsy; they were called latent celiacs. Also classified as latent were a small number who had symptoms of celiac disease that were not confirmed on the initial biopsy but whose endomysial antibodies, when available, were positive. Those who were characterized as potential (pre-celiac) had never had an abnormal biopsy but tested positive when specific antibody testing was done. At least one publication has reported that seven of seven patients who would qualify as potential celiacs developed an abnormal biopsy within one to three years. At the present time, these are not clinically relevant because of the small number of cases but represent the potential expansion of our present thoughts regarding gluten sensitivity by relating the clinical concepts of the disease, the pathological and immunological aspects of gluten-sensitivity, and the clinical scenario of these unusual individuals. When further evidence is available, certain definitions may be changed, and as a result the gluten-free diet may be prescribed for a greater number of people, especially those with positive serological testing regardless of biopsy findings.

A diagnosis of celiac disease and the institution of a gluten-free diet usually means both an answer to what was unexplainable and treatment for the formerly untreatable. The response to this diet is usually rapid, and the prognosis for those correctly diagnosed and treated is excellent. Recent studies have shown that malignancy occurring in those on a gluten-free diet for five years or more is no greater than that of the normal population, as opposed to a prior significant increase in the number of cancer deaths from celiac disease. Their deficiency disorders no longer require supplements, bone problems are resolved, and there is an increased sense of well-being even in those who had few, if any, symptoms. Dermatitis herpetiformis may respond completely, and the diarrhea in diabetics that has previously been ascribed to their basic disease may be resolved. Diabetic control may possibly be more easily managed. Adults with short stature will not grow, but some children respond, and the multiple other associations may correct or become more manageable. There are those who may continue to have diarrhea, with the most common assumption being a failure to follow a gluten-free diet, either overtly or by error. If following reevaluation and correction of their diet they do not improve, further investigation to rule out other causes is indicated. Some of these possibilities are pancreatic insufficiency, lactose or fructose intolerance, intestinal lymphoma or carcinoma, microscopic colitis, an inability to control anal function, or irritable bowel symptoms. A small percent may show no response to either diet or corticosteroids, and these individuals are considered refractory to treatment. These patients can be seriously ill, but recent experience with immunosuppressive drugs in a very few patients has been lifesaving in those instances.

Celiac disease is obviously a much more common disease than reported previously, most likely due to a failure to diagnose. Mass screenings are not only expensive but require enormous effort to carry out properly in order to provide reliable and worthwhile information. On an individual basis, the ability to diagnose or eliminate the possibility of celiac disease is best met by the use of serological screening of those at greatest risk. The absence of the antigliadin antibody will almost entirely eliminate the possibility that celiac disease is present, whereas the presence of this plus the auto-endomysium antibody is 95 to 100 percent positive and indicates the need for a small bowel biopsy. Those who are at the highest risk are the first-degree relatives of patients with known celiac disease, those patients whose complaints or laboratory studies suggest the possibility of celiac disease, and those whose primary disease has been associated with celiac disease.

Some who do not consider the gluten-free diet a lifelong lifestyle may remain well on returning to a regular diet. Regardless, it is, at present, a dictum that for celiacs life without gluten is a lifelong commitment. I believe this is the most difficult dietary regimen to follow because of the multiple uses of gluten and its otherwise hidden presence in the cabinets of family and friends as well as restaurant kitchens. Years ago, compliance was almost an impossible task, but with greater knowledge, greater public and physician awareness, the availability of a large variety of flours, and the presence of different societies and support groups, both cooking and eating have become less complicated; however, celiacs cannot let down their guard. Bette Hagman in this book makes the celiac's life a little easier and eating more exciting as she not only adds new resources and recipes but continues to spread the gospel on how to live with this disorder. Incidentally, these books simplified life for me and I suspect many more physicians who can now confidently recommend her writings rather than explain the dreaded dietary list, that bare-bones description of what you can and can't eat, in a limited period of time. Her work contains not only recipes for foods but those for a full life as well.

Eugene I. Winkelman, M.D., F.A.C.P., F.A.C.G.
Emeritus Physician
Department of Gastroenterology
The Cleveland Clinic Foundation

Preface

When I was asked to revise and update my original *Gluten-free Gourmet* I jumped at the chance since so much progress has been made in the last ten years improving the quality and increasing the availability of gluten-free foods. In the medical field, information and new discoveries about celiac disease and wheat allergies have skyrocketed as well.

I always considered the original book a primer, helping those overwhelmed by the restrictions of the diet to discover how to make enough basic foods that they wouldn't feel deprived. I started developing these recipes because when my doctor told me to eliminate wheat, oats, barley, and rye from my diet, I discovered that the foods I could find were scarce, bland tasting, and/or expensive, but there were no formulas for better ones. I didn't start out to write a book, but, like Topsy, it just grew from a file of my recipes typed to share with other celiacs and, to my surprise, friends who didn't need to avoid gluten but enjoyed the dishes.

As the file grew, I found I had nearly a bookful of tasty ideas to help others avoid the frustrations of watching their companions eat the wheat-laden bread, cake, cookies, and pasta forbidden on our diet. I knew the feeling; I had once suffered it, but now I had developed recipes for all of these, and I wanted to share them.

This revision keeps the book still a primer but it includes a lot of new recipes and revises some of the old using the new flours and added knowledge of the last ten years. At that time rice, whether white or brown, was the basic baking flour. It is mostly starch and has little nutritive value. With the addition of the bean and sorghum flours we have added more nutrition (along with protein) to our baking and can turn out a far more tasty baked product. We've also discovered that our yeast breads are more "batter breads" than the kneaded wheat product and take only one rising. Thus they can be made much more quickly and easily. Bread machines have become household items, and many recipes can be adapted to use this convenience.

This new collection, again, contains very few recipes for plain vegetables, meat, or fruit dishes that one can find in other cookbooks. I concentrated on the baked goods, mixed dishes, and pastas that we usually have to forgo. Although we should be wary of mixed salads when eating out because of the dressings or the pasta or croutons that might be added, we can easily modify most salad recipes to make our own fruit or vegetable combinations.

Since my main concern was to create the best-tasting dishes I could devise using the tricky gluten-free flours, I made no special attempt to keep the recipes low in cholesterol, sodium free, low in calories, or high in fiber. But since many celiacs, especially those newly diagnosed, have a problem with lactose, I tried, whenever possible, to give a choice of a nondairy substitute for a dairy product.

Those who are lactose intolerant may delete the dry milk powder called for in the yeast bread recipes and substitute equal amounts of a nondairy substitute such as Lacto-Free, NutQuik, almond meal, or a powdered baby formula. Each substitute reacts differently and the taste varies. These all contain some protein while other nondairy products contain none. You will achieve a better baked product using those that contain the protein needed to replace the gluten (protein) our flours lack.

Many of these recipes may be further altered to fit other dietetic needs. The diabetic can replace the sugar with special sugar substitutes. For baking, the substitute sugar works best in the heavier, moister cakes (carrot cake, apple-raisin cake, and the like). Those who cannot tolerate soy can replace the soy flour in a recipe with bean or rice flour. (Since soy is more moist, use a bit more liquid.) They should also avoid those nondairy substitutes that are soy based.

If you've never used bean flour before, add it slowly to your diet—

one slice of bread rather than half a loaf a day at first—since beans can cause flatulence in some. Most people adjust well to the bean flours, and they contain necessary B vitamins that rice and the other starchy flours lack.

In some of the recipes, the amount of cholesterol may be lowered by changing the specified meats and cheeses to those with less cholesterol or by using liquid egg substitutes in place of real eggs. You may substitute two egg whites for one whole egg; three egg whites for two eggs. The egg exchange works best in baking if the recipe calls for two eggs or less. In many cases the butter or margarine can be replaced with vegetable oil by reducing the liquid slightly. Remember that in changing a recipe or substituting, you may not achieve the same texture or taste of the original product.

For those who are watching their sodium intake, herbs and spices, light salt, or salt substitute can replace some or all of the salt. Some of the cheeses may be exchanged for varieties lower in sodium.

For those who wish more fiber, it would be easy to substitute brown rice flour for the white in many of the recipes, to add rice bran in some, and to include more high-fiber vegetables in the casseroles and soups.

Many of the cakes, pies, and other desserts are, admittedly, high in calories, but no higher than similar desserts baked with wheat flour. For those counting calories, my only suggestion is to serve smaller portions and, as I do, invite others to share so there will be no leftovers.

Whether you use the recipes as I have written them or alter them to fit other dietary needs, it is my hope that these recipes will make your cooking without gluten tastier and a lot easier.

B.H.

Acknowledgments

This second edition is not mine alone. I could never have written it without the help of many others:

For medical information I appealed to Drs. Joseph Murray of the Mayo Clinic and Alessio Fasano of the University of Maryland School of Medicine. Sam Wylde, Sr., and Sam Wylde III of Ener-G Foods supplied nutritional information, and I owe a great debt to Steve Rice of Authentic Foods for securing the nutritional analyses of all the recipes.

Cynthia Kupper, R.D., CEO of the Gluten Intolerance Group, willingly researched obscure medical data for me and then reviewed the book, correcting errors and rectifying omissions.

One of my greatest debts is to a small group who not only tested the new and revised recipes in a very short time but contributed some of their favorites: Katherine Barkley, Carol Becker, Bert Garman, Marlene Kier, Karen Meyers, Genevieve Potts, Virginia Schmuck, and Mary Lou Thomas. Pam Murray and Nichole Marquette suggested valuable additions.

This book is still *The Gluten-free Gourmet*, and I owe a lot to the original specialists who helped me when I was floundering with both the disease and understanding how to bake with our flours: Jan and Dr. Eugene Winkelman, and Frances Tyus, R.D., L.D., of the Cleveland Clinic Foundation; Gladys Johnson, CSA/USA; and Judy Bodmer, R.D., formerly with Swedish Hospital, Seattle. And most of all to Elaine

Hartsook Ph.D., R.D., founder of the Gluten Intolerance Group, for her years of support and information.

Grateful acknowledgment is made to Judy Lew for the Chinese Corn Soup recipe from her book *Enjoy Chinese Cuisine* (Tokyo, Japan; Joie, Inc., 1984), copyright 1984 by Judy Lew; and to Pat Murphy Garst for her recipe for pizza crust (Pat's Thin Yeast Crust).

The Gluten-free Gourmet

A Diet for Life

When I left my doctor's office over twenty-five years ago clutching three smudged photocopied pages, I was sure that he, like all the other physicians over the years, was just trying to mollify one more skinny hypochondriac. How could a simple diet relieve me of years of bloating, gas, pain, and bouts of diarrhea? I had never heard of nontropical sprue, the term he gave my disease.

One week later I called his office. "You're a genius. I feel better already."

"Just stick to that gluten-free diet and call me back when you start gaining some weight."

By the end of the month I'd read everything I could find (and that wasn't much) about my condition, which had several names: nontropical sprue, celiac sprue, gluten sensitive enteropathy, and, finally, celiac disease. The symptoms were familiar—bloating, diarrhea, backaches, and often just plain stomachache. Others seemed to have constipation with their bloating, and others were only anemic. Another gluten-intolerant condition had symptoms of burning blisters, bumps, or lesions. It has just been in the last decade that those patients with DH (dermatitis herpetiformis) are considered celiacs and put on the gluten-free diet, for, when biopsied, they, too, show damage to the villi. This is really good news for these patients, although they may not consider it so at first, for they can usually reduce their medication slowly and most of them will be able to discontinue it completely as long as they stick to the diet.

I also discovered that I was fortunate in having been diagnosed in the 1970s. Although physicians were aware of celiac disease long before that, until the 1950s there was no answer to what caused the distress symptoms. Many sufferers were limited to eating bananas and rice and were forbidden coarse foods such as other fruits, vegetables, and meat. It wasn't until after World War II that diets could be expanded, when doctors became aware that only the gluten in wheat, barley, rye, and oats was intolerable to patients with celiac disease.

I soon realized, though, that with my improved health and renewed appetite, a diet without wheat, barley, rye, or oats was just plain boring. I didn't mind Cream of Rice for breakfast, but how could I live the rest of my life without bread or pasta or cake or stuffing in my turkey or . . . The list became endless. One day I cheated and ate some freshly baked bread full of the forbidden glutens. The result of that spree was three days in bed suffering the same distress that had sent me to the doctor. I didn't tell him about my slip, but I resolved it would never happen again. Until medical science came up with a better cure for our disease, I'd stick to my diet. I also pledged myself to finding some way to make my food more interesting.

Since I am the kind of noncook who left the plastic wrap on the corned beef the first time I tried boiling it and who had to look up the word *sauté* in the dictionary, I needed help. The health food stores had a couple of boxes of gluten-free baking mix, some rice and soy flours, and Hilda Cherry Hills's book *Good Food, Gluten Free*. Ms. Hills's book contained excellent advice on living, but frankly, the British recipes left me still searching for better taste.

I found an organization called the Gluten Intolerance Group (GIG), which met at our local university school of medicine. Besides providing medical and dietary information, members exchanged cooking hints and recounted horror stories about their own years BD (before diagnosis). I learned I was not alone. In 1990 it was estimated there were over a hundred thousand celiacs in the United States. Even then it was suggested that this may only have been the tip of the iceberg, for many doctors miss the diagnosis—a patient may not recount all his or her symptoms because they sound so diverse. Even more confusing for the patient and the doctor is the fact that celiac sprue symptoms can mimic many other disorders. Very slowly the doctors are becoming more aware of the condition, and in 1997 nationwide blood screening was started for celiac disease. The iceberg is being slowly uncovered. The estimate is running closer to one million celiacs in the United States at this time. With the new and noninvasive blood tests just developed a few years ago, a doctor can screen patients with symptoms first before suggesting the more drastic endoscopy and biopsy. This is now advised for all first- and second-degree relatives of celiacs, for preliminary findings show that approximately 5.7 percent of first-degree relatives and 3.1 percent of second-degree relatives will test positive for the disease. Many of these may have no symptoms as yet, and getting on the diet early may save them from having any of the damaging effects of celiac disease. This damage can cause malabsorption of food and lead to possible anemia, malnutrition, calcium deficiency, mental and/or physical fatigue, or other problems.

I was not aware of any of these possible problems, nor were most people in 1974, but finding that I was not alone with a "rare" disease made me look for more answers. Since then I have joined other celiac groups, become more informed via the increasing amount of literature and medical reports on celiac disease, and have attended national and local conferences in both the United States and Canada. A speaker at one of those conferences described our disease picturesquely: The celiac's immune system mistakes gluten for an enemy and, while fighting it in the gut, flattens or blunts the villi. A healthy villi can be compared to a shag carpet in the intestines soaking up nutrients: the celiac gut resembles linoleum, allowing nutrients to slide unused to the exit.

At the time I was diagnosed, the only flour used for baking was rice, but I soon found that there were other tasty flours we could use: sweet rice, potato, potato starch, soy, tapioca, cornstarch, corn flour, cornmeal, and buckwheat. In the last ten years we've added flours from beans and sorghum, and several of the national organizations recognize that the flours and cereals of amaranth, quinoa, tef, and millet do not contain the toxic gluten. Canada has always considered them gluten-free and allowed them in their celiac diet.

With this wide choice of flours I've discovered it is possible to make good breads, cakes, cookies, and casseroles. I've even baked pizza and lasagne successfully. I stuff my turkey at Thanksgiving and eat plum pudding at Christmas and hot cross buns at Easter. I feed the family and any guests using my diet, and they never suspect they are eating gluten-free foods. In fact, I am often asked for my recipes.

Today the newly diagnosed celiac is more fortunate than I was twenty-five years ago. He or she can join national groups with a chapter nearby, has the choice of more cookbooks, and can find gluten-free bread and mixes in some health food stores or can order, by mail or phone, diet breads, rolls, cookies, gluten-free pasta, and even full main dishes.

Scientists have made progress on the disease, but to date they have not come up with any way other than diet to stop the gliadin factor in gluten from damaging the small intestine. Staying on a gluten-free diet is still the only known way to regain health and remain in remission.

Now I am not even impatient for science to discover some miraculous cure for our disease. With my weight back to normal and my energy high, I eat well within the limitations of the gluten-free diet. I don't think of it as a diet for life, I consider it a prescription for living.

As with any prescription, it has to be filled, and the simplest way to do this is to join a support group—local or national—with a knowledgeable leader. Dieticians and nutritionists are still struggling to understand both cooking with the difficult flours and finding and eliminating hidden gluten, but anyone on the diet soon learns what he/she can have and is more than willing to share at meetings and in the many well-researched newsletters.

There are also two national publications offering information about the disease and a site on the Internet. *Caution:* The Internet has become a sounding board with a lot of information, but this is not monitored so be selective about what you accept when you read it on the screen.

For more information about celiac disease or to find a group near you, contact one of these national organizations:

American Celiac Society Dietary Support Coalition, 59 Crystal Avenue, West Orange, NJ 07052-3570; (973) 325-8837

Canadian Celiac Association, 190 Britannia Road East, Unit 11, Mississauga, Ontario L4Z 1W6, Canada; (905) 507-6208 or (800) 363-7296

Celiac Disease Foundation, 13251 Ventura Blvd., Suite 1, Studio City, CA 91604-1838; (818) 990-2354; fax (818) 990-2397

Celiac Sprue Association/United States of America (CSA/USA), P.O. Box 31700, Omaha, NE 68131-0700; (402) 558-0600

Gluten Intolerance Group of North America (GIG), 15110 10th Avenue, SW, Suite A, Seattle, WA 98166; (206) 246-6652

Internet: http://celiac@maelstrom.stjohns.edu
http://rdz.acor.org/lists/celiac/index.html

References

Ciclitira, P. J., Ph.D., F.A.C.P. (Rayne Institute, St. Thomas' Hospital, London.) "Vision for the Future." Lecture at Celiac Disease Foundation, spring 1992.

Fasano, Alessio, M.D.; Berti, Irene, M.D.; Green, Peter H. R., M.D.; Not, Tarcisio, IRCSS, Garofolo: "Prevalence of Celiac Disease Among First and Second Degree Relatives in the U.S.A." Paper delivered at Digestive Disease Week, Orlando, Florida, 1999.

Hamilton, Helen Klusek, ed. *Professional Guide to Diseases.* Springhouse, PA: Springhouse Corporation, 1987.

Hartsook, Elaine I., R.D., Ph.D. "Celiac Sprue: Clinical Aspects and Patient Realities. What Is Celiac Sprue?" Paper delivered on Celiac Experience I cruise, 1991.

———. "Dermatitis Herpetiformis." Paper delivered at the Gluten Intolerance Group of North America, 1993.

———. "Gluten-Sensitive Enteropathy: Update for Health Care Professionals." Paper delivered at the Gluten Intolerance Group of North America, 1992.

Hopkins, Randy, M.D. "Keeping Your GI Tract in Shape." Lecture at Ballard Hospital Campus, Seattle Center for Digestive Diseases, spring 1994.

Kasarda, Donald, Ph.D. "Celiac Disease." Presentation at North American Society for Pediatric Gastroenterology and Nutrition, Toronto, Canada, October 1997.

Katz, S. "Dermatitis Herpetiformis, The Skin and the Gut." In *Annals of Internal Medicine* 93, no. 6 (December 1980): 857–74.

Murray, Joseph A., M.D. "Celiac Disease in the U.S.A.: Where We Are Vs. Where We Need to Be." Keynote address at annual meeting of the Gluten Intolerance Group of North America, March 1993.

———. "The Widening Spectrum of Celiac Disease." *American Journal of Clinical Nutrition* 69 (1999): 354–65.

Schuffler, Michael. "Medical Facts About Celiac Sprue—New Research." Address to the Gluten Intolerance Group, March 1981.

Seely, Stephen; Freed, David L. J.; Silverstone, Gerald A.; and Rippere, Vicky. *Diet-Related Diseases; the Modern Epidemic*. London and Westport, CT: Croom Helm, AVI, 1985.

Winkelman, Eugene I. "The Many Faces of Sprue." Address at CSA/USA national convention, October 1988.

Zone, John J., M.D. "Dermatitis Herpetiformis." Lecture at annual meeting of the Gluten Intolerance Group of North America, spring 1992.

The Hidden Glutens

I naively assumed when my doctor said no wheat, rye, barley, or oats that I could certainly recognize those, and I mourned the loss of the familiar breads, cookies, and pasta on the grocery shelves. I never dreamed that I would soon be questioning my toothpaste and mouthwash, that I would automatically suspect meats like hot dogs and salami, and that I would learn to ask if there's any filler in my hamburger, "without the bun," of course.

I soon found myself dragging out my magnifying glass on every trip to the grocery store to read labels and was disconcerted to find that gluten had invaded most soups, chilies, and even some of the hash I planned to pick up for that quick-and-easy meal. But it wasn't labeled gluten, nor was it called wheat. Gluten had learned to hide under many labels, and in some instances wasn't labeled at all.

What was even more disquieting was that sometimes a product was gluten free while a lighter form of the product contained gluten and that some products could change formulas from one purchase to the next, so I had to continually keep reading labels.

CANDY

The ingredients in candy must be listed on the label, but currently the companies are not required to list any product that dusts the block the candy is rolled on for shaping. Some candy makers use wheat flour. This was discovered when several celiacs in the Seattle Gluten Intolerance Group complained about symptoms of gluten poisoning after eating candy from a popular local company. The group adviser was told that the ingredients in the candy mixture were gluten free, but as the candy came down the conveyor belt, a dusting of wheat flour was added to make sure the candy would not stick. Thus, the puzzle of the illnesses was solved.

CARAMEL COLOR

Caramel color can be made from dextrose (corn), invert sugar, lactose, molasses, or sucrose (beet or cane). These are gluten free. Caramel color made in the United States and Canada is made from these sources. Imported items containing caramel color can be made from malt syrup or starch hydrolysates, which can include wheat. If in doubt about the caramel color used in an imported food product, contact the company for information.

COFFEE (INSTANT OR POWDERED)

There should be no gluten in powdered coffee, but some flavored coffees may contain the forbidden gluten. Freeze-dried coffee seems less apt to cause problems. If traveling to a foreign country, it's wise to take your instant coffee with you so you are sure to have a familiar brand.

DECAFFEINATED COFFEE

Although the process of decaffeinating should not include the use of glutens, some celiac sufferers have complained of distress on drinking decaffeinated coffee. The culprit could be the chemicals used in the process rather than gluten. Water-processed decaffeinated coffee does not seem to provoke symptoms. The warning about flavored coffee should be observed here, too.

DEXTRIN

This can be made from corn, potato, tapioca, rice, or *wheat.* It is wise to avoid dextrin unless it is labeled as corn dextrin, tapioca dextrin, and so on. To confuse one even more, malto-dextrin is made from cornstarch or potato starch. It is often found in hot dogs, spaghetti sauce, and other such combinations.

ENVELOPES AND STAMPS

Some pastes and glues can contain wheat products. It will not take many licks on an envelope flap that contains a wheat paste before you start feeling distress. To be safe, buy a sponge-topped bottle made for sealing envelopes, fill it with water, and let it do the licking for you. In the last decade, the post office has come out with a wide assortment of self-sticking stamps that require no licking. Then treat yourself to self-sealing envelopes.

FRENCH FRIES

French-fried potatoes made at home or in a restaurant that cooks fresh-cut potatoes in separate oil should be safe, but beware of any place that fries the potatoes in the same hot oil used for breaded products such as fish or chicken. Some of the breading may transfer to the potatoes. Note also that some frozen potato products list wheat on the label.

HYDROLYZED VEGETABLE PROTEIN (HVP) OR HYDROLYZED PLANT PROTEIN (HPP)

These are often found in many canned mixed foods—soups, sausages, and hot dogs—or they could be injected into that holiday turkey. If the label does not tell what this protein is made from, it can be soy, corn, rice, peanuts, or casein from milk or *wheat*. If you wish to use a specific product, you will have to check with the manufacturer to find the source of the HVP or HPP.

IMITATION SEAFOOD

Although imitation seafood (sirimi) starts with a real fish product, a starch binder—cornstarch, potato starch, tapioca flour, or *wheat*—is used to create the look of lobster, crab, or scallops. Be sure to read the label before purchasing this kind of seafood. Even more dangerous to those intolerant of wheat is the tendency in restaurants to mix imitation with real seafood in salads and other dishes. Always ask if there is sirimi in the seafood before ordering a crab, shrimp, or scallop dish in a restaurant or deli.

MODIFIED FOOD STARCH

This is a real bummer! It's listed on food labels from soups to desserts and can be corn, tapioca, or potato starch—all safe. But more frequently it's *wheat*, the most common and least expensive form of thickener for the manufacturer. You'll have to check with him to see what form of starch is used. If the label reads *starch*, in the United States this means cornstarch for foods, but in medications that starch can be corn or wheat. Canadian labels usually read "modified starch" with the derivative in parentheses such as (corn), (tapioca), (potato), and (wheat). A few of the U.S. companies now do this also.

PRESCRIPTIONS AND OVER-THE-COUNTER DRUGS

If you've ever had what appeared to be toxic gluten symptoms after taking a medication ordered by a doctor, you may not have been imagining them. Most tablets, lozenges, and capsules use a filler that can be cornstarch, lactose, or *wheat*. The doctor may be unaware of this or forget to mention it. The wise celiac will check all prescriptions and over-the-counter drugs through his pharmacist. Many times a substitute brand will be gluten free; sometimes a different medication can be prescribed, or in rare cases a pharmacist can compound the drug into a capsule using an acceptable filler.

As for those drugs that use a lactose base, celiacs who are lactose intolerant and suffer bloating, diarrhea, gas, or other distress from this should also look for another brand of drug or try taking the medication with a Lactaid or other lactose-controlling tablet.

RICE SYRUP

This flavoring can contain barley malt and might cause trouble for a celiac. If in doubt about the source of the rice syrup, write to the company for exact information.

TEA

Tea is on the safe drink list for celiacs, but some have complained that instant teas induced discomfort. Again, it could be something else in the powdered product. Remember to read the labels on herb and flavored teas for additives that may contain gluten and always ask for a standard brand of tea, whether iced or hot, when dining out.

TRITICALE AND OTHER SUSPICIOUS GRAINS

Triticale, found in some cereals and some flour mixtures, is a cross of *wheat* and *rye* and is not suitable for a celiac diet. Other grains celiacs should avoid are *bulgur* (wheat that has been boiled, dried, and cracked); *spelt,* an older form of wheat that contains less gluten than the new breeds; *semolina,* the wheat from which much pasta is made; *durum flour,* another name for a hard wheat flour; and *couscous,* a wheat-grain-pasta–like product. For rice couscous products that are acceptable on our diet, see pages 309–15 for suppliers.

For Further Consideration

DISTILLED VINEGAR AND SPIRITS

Canada has always accepted that the distillation process prevents the gluten molecule from ending up in the final product, so they have allowed both distilled vinegar and spirits on their celiac diet list.

In the United States there has been some question, but now most of the celiac organizations are accepting the premise that according to the principles of chemistry *properly distilled* vinegar should not contain any toxic prolamines (fractions of the gluten molecule). In alcohol spirits, for some reason, the scientists have not agreed that a portion of the molecule does not carry over. It is up to the individual to make his or her own decision about whether or not to use either of these products, especially when they are listed as a small percent of the ingredients in condiments or sauces.

Whatever your choice, remember we have rice, wine, apple cider, and other fruit vinegars to use in cooking, and we certainly have enough spirits with tequila, rum, plum and potato vodkas, wines, and brandies that we don't have to feel deprived.

VEINED CHEESE

Roquefort cheese was originally made by rolling bits of French bread into the cheese before putting it into the caves in Roquefort, France, for curing. Today some veined cheeses may use a cultured blue mold. The Dairy Council of Washington stated that the cheese companies would not share their formulas, but they admitted that although the molds are now cultured, they could be of bread origin. Whether these veined cheeses (blue cheese, Stilton, Gorgonzola, and Roquefort) could contain enough gluten to be restricted on a celiac diet is still being questioned.

CONTAMINATION

If you are careful about your diet and think you aren't eating gluten but still feel symptoms, could they be due to contamination? There can be many sources of such contamination in the workplace, environment, during the shipping, handling, and repackaging of gluten-free products. And the greatest of all, the home. Maybe wheat crumbs from the toaster got onto your bread. Did someone whip up a gluten-laced cake or pancakes in the kitchen, leaving the counters white and the air full of flour dust? Look at the cutting board and the butter dish. Are crumbs creeping onto your gluten-free food?

If you bought your rice or other flours at the health food store from a bin next to a gluten flour, maybe the scoops had been exchanged. If the store has a mill attached, check to see if they are milling wheat in the next room. Was the flour you bought ground on stones that had been grinding a gluten flour earlier?

At the workplace, a baker could easily recognize the source of his problems. But a drywall construction person might not realize that the paste he was using contained wheat, which was why he had symptoms after a day of sanding and breathing in the dust.

All these factors and others in your environment must be considered when trying to ferret out the reason for symptoms.

OTHER ALLERGIES AND SENSITIVITIES

If you've eliminated contamination and know you are eating strictly gluten free, then there might be something many doctors and the patients themselves fail to recognize. *It may not be gluten causing the symptoms.* Many celiacs discover they have other allergies or sensitivities they never realized they had until they begin to feel better on the diet. The most obvious is lactose intolerance. That may very well disappear in a short time because the enzyme for digesting lactose is formed on the tip of the villi, and when this regenerates, most patients can return to eating dairy. Some may remain lactose intolerant even after healing. This then appears to be an allergy or sensitivity that has nothing to do with their celiac disease.

Other allergies often discovered (or uncovered) are to eggs, chocolate, shellfish, citrus, peanuts, MSG, corn, and others as wildly diverse as apples or cucumbers. The hardest thing is to single out the food or foods that cause the symptoms. Do this by sticking to a simple diet and monitoring your food. Add foods back into the diet slowly to discover which foods cause distress. The good thing about discovering these is that one can learn to avoid the offending foods, but many find that later the allergies fade and disappear completely, so they can be added back into the diet. The bad thing is that many of the offenders come combined with other foods. Eggs are a part of most baked products, apples come in many mixed juices, while corn can come in several forms from cornstarch to corn syrup to the modified food starch in many products. I've recently heard from readers who are even allergic to rice. The beans, soy, and potato flours have been lifesavers for them.

LEARN TO BE AN EDUCATED LABEL READER

This is a diet for life, but don't expect to learn all the rules the first day. To make it easy on yourself, start with the obvious and work at learning all the hidden sources. Find staples such as mayonnaise, mustard, and ketchup that are gluten free and stick to using those until you feel more confident about the more exotic sauces and seasonings. Many of the support group newsletters frequently contain lists of gluten-free items, and one support group produces a large catalog. In spite of this help, these must be rechecked frequently because companies often change their formulas without any warning.

This sounds like a lot to learn, but slowly you will become an educated, alert, and knowledgeable dieter. Try to be careful, but please don't become paranoid.

References

Bell, Louise; Hoffer, Miriam; and Hamilton, Richard. "Recommendation for Food of Questionable Acceptance for Patients with Celiac Disease." *Journal of the Canadian Dietetic Association,* April 1981.

Campbell, J. A. "Dialogue on Diet." *Celiac News,* Canadian Celiac Association, Ontario, Canada, fall 1990.

Kasarda, Donald, Ph.D. "Plant Toxonomy in Relation to Celiac Toxicity." Presentation at the International Coeliac Symposium, Dublin, Ireland, 1992.

———. "Celiac Disease." Presentation at the North American Society for Pediatric Gastroenterology and Nutrition, Toronto, Canada, October 1997.

Kirshman, Gayla J., *Nutrition Almanac,* 4th ed. New York: McGraw Hill, 1996.

Liston, John. "From Seed to Shining Sea." Address on sirimi at the Institute for Food Science, University of Washington, Seattle, November 1988.

Tyus, Frances J. "Additives . . . Knowing Can Make Your Diet More Flexible." Paper delivered at the National CSA/USA convention, October 1988.

The Gluten-free Diet

It is very difficult to write a diet list for anyone because of other sensitivities and personal preferences. This is a simple list of the foods that those with gluten sensitivity or celiac disease can eat safely and the foods that they should avoid due to the toxic gluten protein found in wheat, rye, barley, oats, and triticale.

Please note that diet regulations vary from country to country. For example, in Canadian celiac organizations, whiskey is on the allowed list even though there is still the question of whether in the distilling process some particles of the toxic gluten carry over into the final product. Wheat starch is allowed in Britain but not in the United States or Canada. Most of the United States celiac organizations now recognize that amaranth, quinoa, millet, and tef do not contain gluten; Canada has always allowed them in the diet. I placed them on neither list since this is a judgment choice that each person will have to make after reading about them on page 44.

This list was compiled from information supplied by my physician, the Gluten Intolerance Group of North America, Mayo Clinic, and the Canadian Celiac Association. I followed the standards of the U.S. organizations.

Foods Allowed	Foods to Avoid
BEVERAGES	
Coffee, tea, cocoa (Baker's, Hershey's, Nestlé), some carbonated beverages, rum, tequila, vodka (if made from potatoes, grapes, or plums), and wine	Postum, Ovaltine, beer, ale, gin, vodka (if made from grain), whiskey, some flavored and instant coffees, some herbal teas, and some carbonated beverages (root beer)
BREADS	
Breads made with gluten-free flours only (rice potato starch, soy, corn, bean, sorghum), baked at home or purchased from companies that produce GF products; rice crackers or cakes, and corn tortillas	All breads made with wheat, oat, rye, and barley flours; all purchased crackers, croutons, bread crumbs, wafers, biscuits, and doughnuts containing any gluten flours; Graham, soda, or snack crackers and tortillas containing wheat
CEREALS	
Cornmeal, hot rice cereals, hominy grits, gluten-free cold rice and corn cereals (those without malt)	All cereals containing wheat, rye, oats, or barley (both the grain and in flavoring, such as malt flavoring and malt syrup)
DAIRY PRODUCTS	
Milk (fresh, dry, evaporated, or condensed), buttermilk, cream, sour cream, butter, cheese (except those that contain oat gum), whipped cream, yogurt (plain and flavored if GF), ice cream (if GF), artificial cream (if GF)	Malted milk, artificial cream (if not GF), some chocolate milk drinks, some commercial ice creams, some processed cheese spreads, flavored yogurt (containing gluten), some light or fat-free dairy products (containing gluten)

DESSERTS	
Any pie, cake, cookie, or other desserts made with GF flours and flavorings; gelatins, custards, homemade puddings (rice, cornstarch, tapioca); prepared cake or cookie mixes (if GF)	All pies, cakes, cookies, etc., that contain any wheat, oat, rye, or barley flour or flavoring; most commercial pudding mixes, ice cream cones, and prepared cake mixes using wheat flour
FATS	
Margarine, vegetable oil, nuts, GF mayonnaise, shortening, lard, and some salad dressings	Some commercial salad dressings and some mayonnaise
FLOURS	
Rice flour (brown and white), soy flour, potato flour, tapioca flour, corn flour, cornmeal, cornstarch, rice bran, rice polish, arrowroot, nut flours, legume, buckwheat, and sorghum flours (see page 44 for amaranth, quinoa, millet, and tef)	All flours or baking mixes containing wheat, rye, barley, or oats
FRUITS AND JUICES	
All fresh, frozen, canned (if GF), and dried (if not dusted with flour to prevent sticking)	Any commercially canned fruit with gluten thickening
MEAT, FISH, POULTRY, AND EGGS	
All eggs (plain or in cooking), all fresh meats, poultry, fish, and other seafood; fish canned in oil, water, or brine; GF-prepared meats such as luncheon meats, tofu, and GF imitation seafood	Eggs in gluten-based sauce, imitation seafood containing wheat flour or gluten flour, prepared meats that contain gluten, some fish canned in HVP, and self-basting turkeys injected with HVP

PASTAS

GF homemade noodles, spaghetti, or other pastas, oriental rice noodles, bean threads, purchased GF pasta made with corn, rice, tapioca, soy, quinoa, and potato flours	Noodles, spaghetti, macaroni, or other pastas made with gluten flours; any canned pasta product

SOUPS AND CHOWDERS

Homemade broth and soups made with GF ingredients, some canned soups, some powdered soup bases, and some GF dehydrated soups	Most canned soups, most dehydrated soup mixes, bouillon, and bouillon cubes containing HVP

VEGETABLES

All plain fresh, frozen, or canned vegetables; dried peas, beans, and lentils	All creamed, breaded, and scalloped vegetables; some canned baked beans and some prepared salad mixes

SWEETS

Jellies, jams, honey, sugar, molasses, corn syrup, syrup, and some commercial candies	Some commercial candies and some cake decorations. Note: icing sugar in Canada may contain wheat.

CONDIMENTS

Salt, pepper, herbs, food coloring, pure spices; rice, cider, and wine vinegars; yeast, GF soy sauce, GF curry powder, baking powder, and baking soda	Some curry powder, some mixed spices, some ketchup, some prepared mustards, and most soy sauces; some pepper with wheat flour added (often found outside the United States)

This is just a general list for your information. Always remember to read the full ingredient list when purchasing any product that might contain any form of gluten.

Raising the Celiac Child

Parents suddenly confronted with the diagnosis of *celiac* for their child may have many conflicting emotions. Sometimes it is relief that they finally found a reason for the child's illness, but this may soon turn to confusion when faced with the diet restrictions. Other times it can be fear that the child may not have a normal childhood. Other emotions are frustration at trying to cook with these different flours and even irritation at the extra time and effort this takes.

One mother admitted to all of these, but the prevailing one was the pleasure of the whole family sharing in the health plan for their daughter (who is now going into her teens with good health). They are all proud that she's well able to choose her own foods, cook many of them, and has educated her teachers, friends, and classmates about celiac disease by serving as an example of a very normal child who has to be careful about what she eats.

It's not going to be easy to convert your food planning from wheat to gluten free but most parents admit that it gets easier as one learns the tricks to make the celiac child never feel deprived or "different."

KEEP A POSITIVE ATTITUDE

1. Be thankful that this condition, unlike many others, is treatable and with proper diet allows for a full life with no medication or painful injections.

2. Whenever possible, make all the main dishes shared by the family gluten free so you have only one meal to prepare and the celiac doesn't feel excluded. This means using the GF Flour Mix for making gravies, stuffing the holiday turkey with a gluten-free dressing, and using the Creamed Soup Base (page 292) for any casseroles. Of course, the celiac can have special bread, cereal, and pasta. Serve it with a gluten-free sauce that all can share. In most cases, the dessert can be a gluten-free one for the whole family to enjoy.
3. Substitute, don't eliminate! If you keep a special box or jar with some treats for the celiac, substitute from this box whenever others are eating wheat treats. Do the same for out-of-home treats at church, school, nursery, or day care. Be sure the caregiver is aware of the box and knows that she should substitute. It will be up to the parent to keep the box filled. Such things as sweet crackers, purchased pretzels, some candy, cookies with a long shelf life, and peanuts are excellent treats. As the child grows and his or her tastes expand, add things like dried fruit snacks and homemade or purchased granola and granola bars.
4. Allow the celiac child to accept social and family affair invitations if the child wishes to go even if it means sending or taking most of the meal and treats for the celiac. It's not easy to learn to cook gluten free, so don't expect family and friends to read all the labels or understand the necessity. If it's a full family meal, take along a dish or two that everyone can enjoy so they'll see that this diet does not have to be dull, tasteless, or boring. Some suggestions are a tasty rice, bean, or potato casserole or a dish such as meatballs, and perhaps add one of the cakes, such as the zucchini or carrot cake. In the casserole use the Creamed Soup Base recipe (page 292) instead of the familiar can of creamed soup. If it's an occasion when only snacks are served, take along enough for others to enjoy of cupcakes or cookies, or prearrange with the hostess to substitute for your child a treat of his/her own in place of the one she is serving.
5. Offer to help. This may not be what you really want to do, but it reinforces your child's positive attitude about the condition when in a care situation. Do this by bringing treats for the whole class or group. Make them all gluten free so your child can join the others

with the same food. You will find other ways of helping once you've started.

6. Offer choices. When I was offered the choice of eating rice cakes or learning to cook, I chose to learn. I'm sure most people would make this choice. The same is true of foods. Don't be afraid to offer a wide variety to eliminate boredom, but be prepared to find that some will be more popular than others and some the child will completely reject. This is the time to watch for other allergies or sensitivities the child may have. Often these are found only when the major intolerance to gluten is controlled; the parent may realize that another food is giving the celiac the same symptoms (see page 15 for allergies and sensitivities).
7. Make it a challenge, not a chore. Your attitude will influence how your child feels about being a celiac. If you keep an upbeat attitude, the child is sure to respond in similar fashion. Since this is a lifelong condition, it's far better for the celiac to start out feeling good about it than to feel depressed or even angry at fate for the rest of his or her life.
8. Join a support group. This should be a priority on your list. You will learn more from others facing the same cooking challenges than from a dietician or nutritionist. You will also find comfort that you are not alone for there will be other parents who are in the same position you are. When possible, take the celiac child along to meet both adults and other children with the same intolerance. (For support groups see pages 6–7.)
9. Get in the habit of planning ahead: *Never leave the house with a hungry celiac and always take a backup snack along.* That tucked-away snack can mean a calm and contented child and a mother who isn't resenting that she can't stop just anywhere to get something. This habit is beneficial for all ages.

THE PRESCHOOL CHILD

It's easy to watch the small child's food in the home, but today's children are exposed to food outside the home: at the nursery school, at play school, and at child care.

Because it is the child who is feeling the symptoms, sometimes it is not possible for a parent or caregiver to recognize that a child has accidentally ingested gluten—whether through a treat, through handling or licking something like play dough or cookie batter, or through the unwitting generosity of one of the workers who feels sorry for the child. In order to avoid these accidents, several suggestions have been made:

1. Pin a badge on the young child with words such as:

I AM ON A SPECIAL DIET
PLEASE DO NOT FEED ME

2. Reinforce this with a letter to be posted on the bulletin board or kept handy that tells all workers that celiac disease is a condition requiring the patient to be on a gluten-free diet because of *damage to the intestines.*

Go on to state simply that all sources of wheat, rye, barley, and oats and their derivatives must be eliminated from the diet. Explain modified food starch, malt and malt flavorings and syrups, and others that might be in foods eaten at the school or home. *Remind them that not even a little bit is okay.*

3. Teach the caregiver to understand labels in order to decide if a purchased snack is safe. This may require a visit to the institution to help the caregiver understand the true nature of the condition. Remind her how easily food may become contaminated. A simple example would be by putting a gluten-free cookie on a plate with gluten-containing cookies. Alert her to nonfood situations such as a texture bin (or sand box) filled with oatmeal.

4. Tell the caregiver what symptoms your child will have, whether it be upset stomach, diarrhea, hyperactivity, change of emotions, or others. This will be a guide to alert her. Note whether you wish to be called when this occurs.

5. Reinforce the positive! Your child is not sick but has a condition that requires only that he or she not eat gluten.

THE ELEMENTARY YEARS

As the celiac child grows, he will gradually take over some of the control of his diet by knowing what to refuse, by learning to read labels himself, and by learning to make his own lunches from the foods he likes to eat at school or other class situations. Thermos bottles of hot soup or main dishes are great. Now that we have good breads, sandwiches can be a change from a hot main dish. Choosing from most cafeteria lines or eating the hot lunches provided at school are seldom satisfactory for the celiac.

During these years it will still be wise to have a written explanation of the disease and the diet to give to the school principal, the secretary, the teachers, and the nurse. It might be helpful if you have a nicely worded one that the child can offer to parents at homes she might visit after school so that the mother won't be offended when your child refuses a treat. Most support groups have a restaurant card that explains this very well. You might want to make copies of your favorite or have the older child carry one (see page 28 for the restaurant card).

What about camp? Several of the celiac organizations offer the camp experience for celiacs. For some the campers will all be celiacs; at others a support group sends volunteer cooks (celiacs themselves) to cook and serve gluten-free meals that are similar to the ones the rest of the campers are eating. To get the latest information on camp locations, dates, and prices call the national organizations listed on pages 6–7.

THE TEENS

It has been noted that many celiacs' symptoms do a disappearing act when they reach their teens. This might make them think the condition has been cured (as doctors formerly thought), but only the symptoms have disappeared, not the disease. So this is a time to be extra careful.

Peer pressure may be great to "come have a pizza" or "have a burger," but even with fast food, the celiac can find a salad that is gluten free or the all-meat burger without the bun. And in some places the french fries are fried separately, so they will be gluten free (if the restaurant doesn't dust them first with wheat flour). Joining the others for a Coke will still give the celiac a chance to "hang out" with friends.

The most important thing about keeping the teenage celiac from cheating is to have plenty of substitutes for those appealing gluten-filled snacks and treats. A freezer packed with gluten-free goodies at home would certainly deter the celiac from reaching for a gluten-laced product.

LEAVING HOME

The young adult celiac leaving home for college or first shared apartment is forced to face the diet either without a kitchen or (at best) sharing a limited space. This will mean resorting to buying bread or learning to use a bread machine. The very first thing a celiac will note is that he'd better acquire some basic cooking skills.

There are suppliers of baked breads, cake, and cookies, and many offer mixes for these staples. Some can be found on health food store shelves and, hopefully, soon will be on regular grocery shelves. There are also suppliers who ship whole meals frozen, and others offer dried main dishes suitable for camping and hiking because it takes only boiling water to reconstitute them. These are costly but in emergencies could supplement the fresh fruits, vegetables, meats, and eggs served on campus or cooked in that first apartment. Other quick meals could center around gluten-free canned hash or chili, or canned or dried gluten-free soups.

The choices may seem limited, especially if on a budget, but the celiac will not even have to forgo pizza because some suppliers offer frozen or dry pizza shells that most pizza parlors will be willing to fill with one's choice of toppings.

One of the biggest problems some celiacs face is finding that their housemates are snacking from the celiac's carefully hoarded supplies. Solving this is going to take tact and diplomacy. With determination, the right attitude, and "care" packages from home the young adult celiac can even survive these difficult years.

A final reminder: No matter at what age your child is diagnosed, try to convince all first-degree relatives—siblings, parents, and grandparents—to take the noninvasive blood screening test. Since the first results of nationwide screening are proving that these relatives are at a higher risk of having the disease than the general public, this just might turn up another celiac in the family, one who has no symptoms yet and is unaware of the damage being done to the body already.

Reference:

Berti, Irene, M.D.; Karoly Horvath, M.D.; Peter H. R. Green, M.D.; Tarcisio Not, IRCSS; Burlo Garofolo; Alessio Fasano, M.D. "Prevalence of Celiac Disease Among First and Second Degree Relatives in the U.S.A." Paper delivered at Digestive Disease Week, New Orleans, Louisiana, 1999.

Traveling and Eating Out

Eating out on our diet may seem at first an exercise in frustration, with all those delectable dishes on the menu that we can't order. But just as the diabetic learns to avoid sugar and the overweight person shuns the high-calorie dishes, the celiac learns to recognize gluten.

It's easy to wave away the bread and to refrain from ordering pasta, breaded or stuffed meats, or casserole dishes, but from there on the menu should be discussed with the serving person or chef. Is the steak marinated in a sauce that could contain gluten before being broiled? Is the liver or other meat floured before grilling? Does the salad contain croutons, and the salad dressing wheat? Was the turkey stuffed before roasting, or was the stuffing baked separately? Is the soy sauce in that Chinese dish made from wheat or soy?

Twenty-five years ago, as a newly diagnosed celiac, I was embarrassed to ask questions that might send my waitress or waiter back to the kitchen several times, and as a result I often received food that I had to leave untouched. Now I ask as I pull from my wallet my handy restaurant card. Most of the celiac organizations offer one of these, but the one I use is the most official looking, plasticized, and the size of a credit card. (It is available from the Gluten Intolerance Group; see page 7.) It has a simple explanation for the server or chef:

> It is IMPERATIVE that persons with this hereditary disorder avoid eating: WHEAT, RYE, OATS, BARLEY and all derivatives

of these grains to avoid intestinal damage. Other sources include: flour thickeners, coating mixes, sauces, soy sauce, marinades, malt, malt flavoring, hydrolyzed vegetable protein, modified food starch, pasta, croutons, stuffings, some herbal teas, broth, self-basting poultry and imitation bacon, seafood and soup base.

Since this explanation is short and easily read, most serving people have been obliging, sometimes bringing the cook to the table or taking me to the cook. I give the restaurant four stars in my book when the cook understands and makes me a plate that looks great, tastes great, and is completely gluten free. And the cook gets five stars when others in the restaurant look at my plate and wonder where I found *that* on the menu.

If the cook finds the restaurant card daunting, it's still easy for him to prepare a good meal if you suggest grilled or plain roasted (no "au jus" or bouillon-basted) meat, or grilled or poached fish, with potatoes (parsley-buttered or baked), and some plain vegetable or fruit.

Another trick is to look at the appetizer list. What's wrong with stuffed potatoes or clams in their own broth or an avocado stuffed with seafood (as long as there's no sirimi in it) or a serving of potato skins with cheese and bacon bits as a main course? If you have taken along your crackers or, better yet, some of the bread sticks you'll find on pages 63 and 64, you won't envy your dinner companion that chicken-fried steak, stuffed pork chop, or even the crusty breaded oysters.

This is simple for you if the restaurant has a full menu, but even fast-food places can provide a good meal. I've ordered a "sandwich" without the bread and had a full serving of ham or turkey with lettuce and tomato or cheese. When ordering soup to go with it, I make sure it doesn't contain barley or pasta, have a wheat thickener, or start with a bouillon cube. Try hamburgers without the bun, french fries, and salads at McDonald's or head for the salad bar at the nearest pizza parlor.

If all else fails, turn to the breakfast menu. An omelet tastes good anytime, and one stuffed with meat and vegetables can be a full meal.

These are only a few suggestions to get you over those first visits to a restaurant. You'll probably find after a short time that any eating establishment can provide a good gluten-free meal with a few suggestions from you and an obliging cook.

TRAVEL IN THE UNITED STATES

The rules above can be followed for any eating out, whether for a single meal or while traveling, but for anything longer than a day trip you might want to pack a "survival kit." For me this is a supply of crackers and granola bars, cheese (single slices wrapped separately), dried or fresh fruit, cookies, and some candy. You can add some granola or muesli to tide you over when all that's offered is a continental breakfast. I have carried this kit on a train through China, and it has helped me survive long plane trips, bus excursions, and even a breakdown in the British midlands.

By far the best way for the celiac to vacation is camping, where you carry and cook your own food, whether you rough it in a tent or travel by trailer or motor home. When you go to a resort, rent a condo rather than a hotel room and eat some meals in.

For more extensive traveling, the cruise ship is the easiest on our diet. Take along a few of your breads and cookies, and talk over your diet with the maître d' as soon as you go aboard. If there is no refrigerator in your stateroom, he will put your food in one of the kitchen refrigerators, and your waiter will bring items out as needed. If you carry along a few of your own mixes, the chef will have these made up for you to have fresh muffins, bread, or cake on the cruise. I always keep a supply of granola bars and crackers in my stateroom either for snacks or for taking with me when we leave the ship for a day's shore excursion.

Eating on planes can be a bit trickier. Although almost all the airlines now offer a supposedly gluten-free meal (they weren't even available ten years ago), some of the airline kitchens do not understand what gluten free means. On my last trip I was served the vegetarian meal (pasta) with a diabetic twist (all the sugar removed). Since I always carry a small survival packet in my purse or carry-on, I dug that out and had a satisfactory snack while the gluten-laden spinach pasta withered in front of me. But always order the gluten-free meal; many times they are gluten free (unless the stewardess thinks the tray looks too bare and adds one of the wheat rolls as a finishing touch). *Warning:* Be wary of any bread, rolls, or cookies that are not wrapped and therefore do not have the ingredients listed on the label.

If you're like me, you may be the only one on the cruise or tour with a larger container for your food than you have for your clothes. If you are planning to join a guided excursion where luggage is limited, it would be wise to write ahead to the company and ask permission for this extra box or suitcase. Include the name, number, and date of your tour.

TRAVELING ABROAD

The suggestions above can help make even foreign travel easier. For foreign travel, your packet of extras could include dried soups, canned tuna and chicken, a small jar of peanut butter, and some of the freeze-dried foods provided for backpackers and campers. Most foreign hotel rooms provide a hot kettle or hot water so you can easily make a cup of soup and have a cracker sandwich to go with it. Add a sweet, and you're ready to go exploring. You won't be the only one doing this. Many experienced travelers have learned these tricks to save time, money, and disappointment when they discover they've reached a hotel ten minutes after the dining room closed.

There are a few other factors to be considered when going abroad. Most countries do not restrict the celiac diet to zero tolerance as do Australia, Canada, and the United States. If you buy a product labeled gluten free in other countries, it may contain .3 percent protein (possibly gluten), and they allow wheat starch to be used in their baked products. The United States and Canada discontinued the use of wheat starch in the 1970s because of the trace of gluten residue. If you are offered gluten-free breads abroad, look at the label or ask to see the ingredient list to be sure you aren't being served a product made with wheat starch. Reading that label will take a bit of translating. Their *corn flour* is equivalent to our modified food starch (which can be wheat, corn, or another flour); *maize flour* is their corn flour, while *wheaten corn flour* is definitely wheat flour.

WHAT TO CARRY BESIDES THE FOOD

When traveling to countries that do not read or speak English, you can order the card I mentioned earlier in several languages, but I have a few simple lines that I often have my guide or a souvenir shopkeeper translate into the local language:

I do not speak your language. I have celiac disease. If I eat any food containing even a trace of wheat, rye, oats, or barley, I will become ill. If necessary, please check with the chef to be sure my food does not contain any of those ingredients and help me order a meal I can safely eat.

Thank you very much!

Some countries do not allow you to bring in any food. To avoid having your survival box confiscated at a border, carry a letter signed by your physician saying you need this food. I keep mine tucked in my passport because it's the customs and immigration official who will ask if you are bringing food into the country. You might want to mark your food box or bag with the words *Medical Supplies*.

If you follow these few suggestions, eating out while traveling can be easy. And as a bonus, when the food is gone, there will be extra space in your luggage for those souvenirs.

A TRIP TO THE HOSPITAL

A trip you often cannot plan is one to a hospital. Eating gluten free there is going to take some explaining on your part and (sometimes) help from friends on the outside. In spite of all the advances in the last few years, many hospitals are not equipped to furnish gluten-free meals, so you will have to describe exactly what you can and cannot have. This is another place the restaurant card comes in handy. If you have a chance and your stay is planned, go to the hospital ahead of time and talk to the dietician, but remember to have your doctor put the order on your chart.

Always be sure you ask about every medication. You don't want to be surprised by a filler of gluten in a pill the nurse hands you to "make you feel better." You can request an "allergy" armband marked "No gluten." These must be checked before any medications or foods are given.

If your stay is to be very long, you might be wise to cook up a few casseroles and freeze them in one-meal servings or order from the suppliers some of the frozen main dishes now offered. Have a friend or spouse bring these when visiting. They're sure to be more welcome than flowers.

Time- and Money-Saving Tips for the Cook

The gluten-free diet is going to seem overwhelming at first. There is so much to learn and so many different flours and unusual additives that both the pocketbook and the brain are challenged. Don't be discouraged; just take it one step at a time. Ask for help from other celiacs in a support group and send for the supplies you can't buy locally from the many suppliers listed in the back of this book. You can find some mixes to start you out and even some full meal items.

Although there are a lot of foods you can and will order, many celiacs find it much less expensive and the food tastier when they cook their own bread, cake, cookies, and even pasta. Cooking from scratch, as you will discover, takes extra time, but there are shortcuts to make it easier.

Buy baking ingredients in quantity and stir up your own mixes. This applies to both flour mixes and mixes for muffins, waffles, and bread. On pages 38–39 you will find two flour mixes I use in many of my baking recipes. I always keep these on hand in large canisters. I also double or triple the amount of dry mixture for my breads and keep these stored (in tightly sealed plastic bags) for another baking, thus saving time and mess on a future day.

Do not add the yeast until baking day. For pancakes, muffins, and biscuits, the dry ingredients can be mixed ahead of time and stored, needing only the addition of eggs, liquid, and oil at the last minute.

Use as many prepared foods as possible. Many frostings, sauces, and seasoning mixes are safely gluten free, but always remember to check the ingredient list to be sure they haven't changed formulas since the last time you purchased them. There are rice and corn pastas available on the grocery shelves, or order excellent pastas from the suppliers with a simple phone call (see the list on pages 309–15).

Keep the Creamed Soup Base (page 292) *near your stove.* This makes the equivalent of one can of creamed soup (chicken or mushroom) in just a minute or two.

Make as much of the meal gluten free as possible so you don't have to make two main dishes, salads, or desserts. Gluten free can be both healthy and tasty, so the family won't suffer. Since gluten-free pasta is time consuming to make and expensive to buy, the cook might want to boil separate pasta for the celiac but make a sauce everyone can eat.

Buy, instead of making, gluten-containing cookies and bread in order to avoid contamination in the kitchen and the air, thus forcing more cleanup.

Save all stale GF bread or baking mistakes. These were expensive to make, so use them for stuffing and casseroles, or dry them in the oven and turn them into crumbs with a food processor or blender. Freeze them to use later in crumb crusts for pies and cheesecakes. If you want them to taste like graham cracker crumbs, add a bit of cinnamon and sugar.

Make gravies the whole family can enjoy using the GF Mix (page 38). Just use this as you would any wheat flour by browning in the drippings and adding water to achieve a thick gravy; thin with water or milk (or nondairy liquid) to the desired consistency.

When baking and the recipe calls for crushed GF cereal, crush it in a plastic bag. Roll with a rolling pin and then, if you are using the cereal as a piecrust, add the melted margarine or butter and sugar to the cereal in the bag and blend by shaking. Dump into the pie tin and pat out. No bowl to clean.

Freeze single portions of GF leftovers on small microwavable frozen food trays or in freezer containers. Pull these out for the gluten-intolerant diner when a dish containing gluten is served to the rest of the family.

Keep a good supply of rice or corn crackers on hand. The small, round Asian ones are great for hors d'oeuvres or snacking. *Always read the ingredient list because some of these have gluten in the seasoning.* There are several thin crackers on the grocery shelves that could make sandwiches and are great for carrying when dining out or shopping. They can also be crushed and used as crumbs for baking. Many of the suppliers also carry crackers. Order several boxes to keep handy when the bread box is bare.

The microwave, freezer, food processor, and heavy-duty mixer save work and time. They are well worth the investment. Many celiacs use a bread machine for mixing and baking their bread. (See pages 51–52 for information on bread machines.) Some recipes in this book are written for both hand mixing and the bread machine.

Buttermilk for baking (and many GF recipes call for this) *can be kept on hand.* Store a can or box of powdered buttermilk on the kitchen shelf and then reconstitute when making up the recipe—or see the substitution list below.

If you don't have an ingredient, try an emergency substitute. In many cases you don't have to dash off to the grocery store to find a recipe item if you use one of the following substitutions:

1 square chocolate = 3 tablespoons cocoa + 1 tablespoon butter
1 cup buttermilk = 1 cup yogurt
1 cup milk = ½ cup evaporated milk + ½ cup water
1 cup sour milk = 1 cup milk + 1 tablespoon lemon juice or vinegar
1 cup sugar = 1 cup honey (use ¼ cup less liquid in recipe)
1 teaspoon baking powder = ¼ teaspoon baking soda + ½ teaspoon cream of tartar
1 cup brown sugar = 1 cup granulated sugar
1 cup oil = 1 cup (2 sticks) butter or margarine
1 tablespoon prepared mustard = 1 teaspoon dry mustard
1 clove garlic = ⅛ teaspoon garlic powder

Check this equivalent chart before you start a recipe to be sure you have enough of an ingredient:

Bread crumbs: 1 slice bread = ½ cup crumbs
Cheese: 1 pound cheese = 4 cups shredded or grated
Butter or margarine: 2 sticks = 1 cup
Herbs: 1 teaspoon dried = 1 tablespoon fresh
Pasta and rice:

Macaroni: 1 cup uncooked = 2½ cups cooked
Noodles: 1 cup uncooked = 1 cup cooked (or slightly more)
Rice: 1 cup = 3 cups cooked

Replacements: In many cases one item of food can easily replace another in the recipe, such as:

Raisins for dried cranberries
Golden raisins in place of raisins or currants
Dried orange or lemon peel for orange or lemon zest: 1 teaspoon dried peel = 1 tablespoon zest
Nuts can be used interchangeably, but the flavor will be different. Almonds are mild, macadamia nuts are very fatty, while pecans and walnuts interchange well.

Gluten-free foods are getting better and more varied as the number of vendors grows. Our specialty foods may become more easily available at the local health food store and even on grocery shelves, so you may not have to become the supercook as we did in the last decade. Ask your supermarket managers to stock specific products in their stores and thank them when they do. With more celiacs being diagnosed and more awareness, we may not remain the starving orphans of the food supply chain.

Cooking with Gluten-free Flours

The first baking I tried with gluten-free flours produced a powdery, tasteless muffin that even my ever hungry grandson rejected. I ate the thing because I was hungry for a bread substitute. Actually, I licked it from my cupped hand because it was mostly crumbs. One of the next things I tried to bake was bread using a wheat recipe and merely substituting rice flour. What I created was a brick that might have broken my toe if I had dropped it. My poodle gnawed at it a bit and then decided the only sensible thing to do was bury it.

A lot has changed since those first attempts. I've learned the secrets of working with these weird-acting flours. And over the years my foods have gotten better. In fact, they are now so good that I have to remind my wheat-eating friends: "Hey! Leave some for me." Gluten-free flours made from rice, beans, or tapioca take a bit of pampering, but your baked products can taste as good as the wheat ones you may only dimly remember—if you follow a few simple rules:

1. Because the flours do not contain gluten, the "stretch" factor, baked products tend to be dry and crumbly unless some other stretch factor is added. This can be extra egg white, cottage or ricotta cheese, unflavored gelatin, extra leavening, a product called Egg Replacer (not an egg product), and the addition of xanthan or guar gum.
2. Flours without gluten produce better products when used in combination. One can use white rice flour plus tapioca for a fine-textured

cake; brown or white rice flour plus potato starch and tapioca in breads; rice flour plus soy in fruit-filled cakes or waffles; and potato starch flour plus cornstarch in pizza dough. This blending of flours is probably much like the various wheat flours blended by mills for different uses. This also holds true for the new flours, bean and sorghum. Although they contain more protein than rice flour and make more wheatlike products, they need to be blended also.

Two of the blends I've used in this book both equate with wheat flour in recipes and often can be used interchangeably, although the texture of the finished product may be quite different.

FLOUR MIXES AND HOW TO USE THEM

Gluten-free Mix: This will be referred to as GF Mix in the recipes. This is the original mix I developed. It is a heavy mix and leaves a slightly grainy taste in the baked product, but the mix exchanges cup for cup with wheat flour in adapting recipes. Because of its low protein count, you must add extra protein and/or leavening (egg whites, dry milk powder or a nondairy substitute, gelatin, or Egg Replacer).

FORMULA:	FOR 9 CUPS:
2 parts white rice flour	**6 cups white rice flour**
⅔ part potato starch flour	**2 cups potato starch flour**
⅓ part tapioca flour	**1 cup tapioca flour**

Four Flour Bean Mix: This new combination I formulated recently may revolutionize gluten-free baking. Not only does this exchange cup for cup with wheat flour, but it has enough protein so that in many cases you can take your regular cake or cookie recipe and not have to make any additions except for some xanthan gum. *Always remember to introduce bean flour into your diet slowly since beans can cause flatulence in some people for a short time.*

FORMULA:	FOR 9 CUPS:
⅔ part Garfava bean flour	**2 cups Garfava bean flour**
⅓ part sorghum flour	**1 cup sorghum flour**
1 part cornstarch	**3 cups cornstarch**
1 part tapioca flour	**3 cups tapioca flour**

You can mix these yourself or order them premixed from some of the suppliers listed on pages 309–15. Both have a long shelf life and may be stored at room temperature. Even though these equate with wheat flour, you will have to do a bit more to convert that favorite recipe to gluten free. Often a little extra egg and leavening along with xanthan gum will turn out a satisfactory product. A basic formula for using xanthan gum (necessary with all gluten-free flours) is:

For breads: ¾ teaspoon per cup of flour
For cakes: ½ teaspoon per cup of flour
For cookies: ¼ to ½ teaspoon per cup of flour

If you haven't worked with these flours before, it's easiest to start with simple recipes to satisfy the craving for something besides rice crackers, but it won't be long before you can turn out baked products that nondieting friends will enjoy as well. As a thickening agent, I use the GF Mix in all my gravies, potato starch and sweet rice flour in cream sauces and soups, and tapioca and cornstarch in pies and fruit dishes.

If you live at a high altitude, you should follow your usual adjustments for the altitude including the changes made in oven temperatures. If you have questions, your local county extension agent will have the correct measurements for your location.

PRINCIPLES OF SUBSTITUTION

All the flours have a different absorptive value, and though it is best to follow the recipes in gluten-free cookbooks as written when first working with gluten-free flours, if you want to experiment, you can try to substitute for 1 cup of wheat flour as follows:

1 cup GF Mix
1 cup Four Flour Bean Mix
⅞ cup rice flour
⅝ cup potato starch flour
1 cup soy flour plus ¼ cup potato starch flour
½ cup soy flour plus ½ cup potato starch flour
1 cup corn flour
1 scant cup fine cornmeal

You've probably used few of these flours before, so here's a short explanation of what each is and how best to cook with and store them. I've also included some of our unusual baking additives:

ARROWROOT

This white flour is ground from the root of a West Indian plant and can be exchanged measure for measure with cornstarch in recipes and mixes if you are allergic to corn. I do not call for this in any recipe in this book.

GARBANZO BEAN FLOUR

Ground from garbanzo beans (often called chickpea or cici beans), this flour may be used in combination with Romano bean flour (equal parts) to make a flour similar to the Garfava flour. Do this if you are allergic to fava beans.

GARFAVA FLOUR

This smooth combination of garbanzo and fava beans, produced by Authentic Foods (see suppliers, page 310), is a staple in many of my recipes. It is high in protein and nutrients and makes a better textured baked product than rice flour. The flour is very stable and may be stored in the pantry. See Garbanzo Bean Flour if you are sensitive to fava beans.

ROMANO BEAN FLOUR

A dark, strong-tasting bean flour, this is milled from the Romano or cranberry bean. The flour is high in fiber and protein, and can be used in combination with Garbanzo Bean Flour to make a flour similar to Garfava Flour (see above). It can be purchased in health food stores in Canada and from mail-order suppliers in the United States.

BUCKWHEAT FLOUR

Canada has always allowed this flour in the GF diet. Only recently have most of the United States organizations agreed that in spite of its unfortunate name, the flour is not related to wheat but to rhubarb. Because of its strong taste, it is more easily accepted when used in small amounts to give flavor to other bland flours. Start using it by trying a tablespoon or two in pancakes or waffles if you wish to include it in the diet.

CORNSTARCH

This refined starch from corn is used in combination with other flours to make one of my baking mixes. If allergic to corn, replace this with arrowroot in mixes and recipes.

CORNMEAL

This meal, ground from corn, may be obtained in yellow and white forms. Combine this with other flours for baking or use it alone in Mexican dishes.

CORN FLOUR

A flour milled from corn, this can be blended with cornmeal when making corn breads and corn muffins.

NUT FLOURS

Chestnut, almond, and other nut flours can be used in small quantities, replacing a small portion of other flours to enhance the taste of homemade pasta, puddings, and cookies. I haven't included any recipes in the book, but chestnut flour can be added to your pasta mix and to plain cake mixes. Since they are high in protein, nut flours are a great addition to the diet if you have the opportunity to experiment.

POTATO STARCH FLOUR

Made from potatoes, this fine white flour is used in the Gluten-free Mix. This keeps well and can be bought in quantity.

POTATO FLOUR

Do not confuse this with potato starch flour. This is a heavy flour. Buy it in small quantities because you will need very little of it. Store in the refrigerator.

WHITE RICE FLOUR

This very bland (and not very nutritious) flour milled from polished white rice doesn't distort the taste of any flavorings used. It has long been a basic in gluten-free baking, but the more nutritious bean flours are now gaining popularity. This can be stored in the pantry and has a long shelf life.

BROWN RICE FLOUR

This flour, milled from unpolished brown rice, contains bran and is higher in nutrient value than white rice flour. Use it for breads, muffins, and cookies where a bran (or nutty) taste is desired. Because there are oils in the bran, it has a much shorter shelf life and tends to become stronger tasting as it ages. Purchase fresh flour and store it in the refrigerator or freezer for longer life.

SWEET RICE FLOUR

This flour, made from a glutinous rice often called "sticky rice," is an excellent thickening agent. It is especially good for sauces that are to be refrigerated or frozen because it inhibits separation of the liquids. I also add it by the tablespoon to breads in my bread maker when the dough is too thin. I've found this in many grocery stores under the label Mochiko Sweet Rice Flour, but it can be ordered from several of the suppliers or found in some Asian markets. Do not confuse it with plain white rice flour.

RICE POLISH

This is a soft, fluffy, cream-colored flour made from the hulls of brown rice. Like rice bran, it has a high concentration of minerals and B vitamins. And like rice bran, it has a short shelf life. Buy this at a health food store and keep it in the freezer or refrigerator.

SORGHUM FLOUR

This new flour ground from specially bred sorghum grain is available from several suppliers and should soon be on the shelves of some health food stores. This combines with the bean flours to make my Four Flour Bean Mix, which is used in many recipes in this book. Sorghum flour is seldom used alone. It stores well on the pantry shelf. Sorghum flour also sells under the names milo and jowar.

SOY FLOUR

A yellow flour with high protein and fat content, this has a nutty flavor and is most successful when used in combination with other flours in baked products that contain fruit, nuts, or chocolate. Purchase it in small quantities and store in the freezer or refrigerator because it, too, has a short shelf life. Some celiacs may be sensitive to this flour. Bean flour can be substituted in many recipes that call for soy.

TAPIOCA FLOUR

Made from the root of the cassava plant, this light, velvety white flour imparts "chew" to our baked goods. I use it in both my mixes. It can be stored at room temperature for a long time.

Some Flours That Have Been Questioned

AMARANTH, QUINOA, MILLET, AND TEF

These four flours, more exotic and less well known, have been accepted in Canada for years as gluten free. Most of the United States groups are coming to accept the fact that botanically they are not connected to the gluten-containing grains, but all emphasize that one should watch out for contamination in growing, shipping, and handling. As with all flours, there is always the chance that a person will be allergic or sensitive to one or another. Since these have not been a staple of the diet here, introduction of any of these grains is best made slowly. An understanding of their botanical relatives may help to determine whether you want to try these flours, which have a nutritive value far surpassing that of rice.

Amaranth flour is ground from the seed of a plant related to pigweed.

Quinoa seeds come from a plant in a family related to spinach and beets. These grow with a bitter coating, so always buy debittered flour.

Millet and Tef (Teff) are grains in the same grass family as corn, rice, and sorghum.

Flours on the Restricted List

SPELT, KAMUT, CLUB, DURUM, BULGUR, EINKORN, AND SEMOLINA

These are all different species of wheat and should be eliminated in any form from the gluten-free diet.

TRITICALE

This is a hybrid of rye and wheat. Not for a gluten-free diet!

OATS

Some medical experts are now listing oats as only "possibly" containing toxic gluten, but most doctors in the United States don't want to commit their patients to oats in the diet at this time. Whether people on a gluten-free diet can safely eat oat products remains a subject of scientific debate. Difficulties in identifying the precise amino acids responsible for the immune response and the chemical differences between wheat and oats have contributed to the controversy.

Other Baking Supplies

XANTHAN GUM

This is a powder milled from the dried cell coat of a microorganism called *Xanthomonas campestris*, grown under laboratory conditions. It replaces the gluten in yeast breads and other baking with our flours. It is available in some health food stores and by order from some of the suppliers listed on pages 309–15.

GUAR GUM

A powder derived from the seed of the plant *Cyamopsis tetragonoloba*, this powder can be purchased in health food stores or ordered from suppliers. Because it has a high fiber content and is usually sold as a laxative, it can cause distress in people whose digestive systems are sensitive. This can be used in place of xanthan gum in baking.

DRY MILK POWDER

I used to call for nonfat, non-instant milk powder in my recipes until some readers complained that they were sensitive to so much milk powder. Now I suggest that you can use the regular powder from your grocery. This will still turn out excellent bread and baked products.

NONDAIRY POWDERED MILK SUBSTITUTES

The lactose intolerant can substitute either Lacto-Free or Tofu White (both contain soy), NutQuik (made from almonds), or almond meal for the dairy milk powder. Another choice could be one of the powdered baby formulas from the supermarket or drugstore. Some are soy based and other corn.

LIQUID EGG SUBSTITUTES

These cholesterol-free liquid substitutes for whole eggs are made from the egg whites plus other ingredients. They may be found in the dairy section and freezer cases of most grocery stores. *Always read the ingredient labels to be sure the one you choose doesn't contain gluten or some other ingredient to which you are allergic.*

EGG REPLACER

This powdered substitute for eggs in cooking contains no egg product and is also free of dairy, corn, soy, and gluten. I use a little of this for extra leavening in many recipes. Egg replacer can be ordered from Ener-G Foods or found in most health food stores. A similar product is also available in Canada.

DOUGH ENHANCERS

These powdered products are used in bread making to substitute for the vinegar that balances the pH in most waters. They also tend to make the bread stay fresh longer. They are produced by many companies and can be found in baking supply stores and some health food stores. *Always read the ingredient labels to find one that's gluten free and doesn't contain anything else to which you may be sensitive.* Several suppliers listed on pages 309–15 carry dough enhancers.

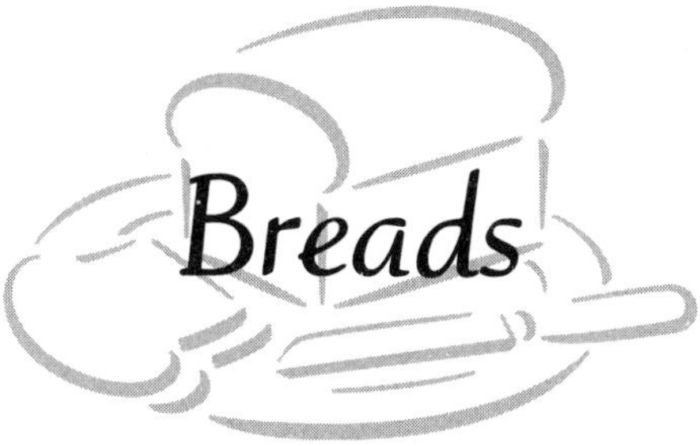

Breads

Small Breads

See Also

I'm sure my fellow celiacs dream, as I do, of the time when we can walk into any grocery store and buy a loaf of fresh gluten-free bread. Unfortunately, this is still in the dream stage, but there is promise that in the near future we will be able to either buy bread in the freezer section or pick up a mix from the shelf. There are a lot of suppliers who sell bread by mail order and others who sell mixes, but none of these products can compare to the absolute joy of taking fresh hot loaves of bread from the oven or a bread machine.

This bread can be light and chewy now for one of the greatest advances in the last ten years is in the making and baking of gluten-free breads. A decade ago our basic bread, made of rice, took four hours to make and came out heavy and gritty tasting, and all too often it crumbled into our laps. Today our breads are easy to make, springy to the touch, and delicious to eat with no crumbling. We've come a long way!

When I first started baking gluten-free bread, I followed the rules for wheat bread by allowing two kneadings and an extra rising before finally spooning the dough into pans and placing them into the oven. I've learned a lot since then. All the bakers working with gluten-free flours pooled their findings to discover that our dough does not require this double treatment because the yeast is not reacting to gluten and has little to feed on in the second rising. The double rising turns out a much denser loaf of bread than the single rising. Simple, isn't it?

Since I've found how easy gluten-free bread is to make, I usually use the hand-mixing and oven-baking method and have my bread finished in about 1½ hours. This allows more control over the rising and baking time and turns out a lighter, finer-textured loaf. I can also choose the size and shape of loaf I want. This control is seldom possible when using a bread machine.

If you are not familiar with baking bread, there are a few simple rules that will help ensure success:

Do not attempt to use a wheat flour recipe and substitute gluten-free flour.

Follow the mixing directions carefully.

Always check the date on the yeast package to be sure your yeast is fresh.

Let bread rise in a warm place. Find a draft-free corner of the kitchen or bath.

Use lukewarm water only. Hot water will kill the yeast; cold water will prevent it from working. Test with a thermometer (105°–115°) or put a drop on the inside of your wrist as one tests milk for a baby's bottle.

Use a heavy-duty mixer (such as a KitchenAid) to beat the bread. The dough is softer and stickier than gluten bread dough and cannot be kneaded by hand.

Use xanthan gum for all the yeast recipes to make the breads springy. It replaces, in part, the gluten that rice, potato, and bean flours lack.

Substitute guar gum for xanthan gum in equal amounts, if necessary, but guar gum, often sold as a laxative, may cause distress to some who eat the bread.

Always use the size pans called for in the recipe.

On days of high humidity, increase the amount of yeast by ½ to 1 teaspoon. This will help the bread rise faster. Do this for hand mixing only.

Use brown rice flour for extra nutrition or a combination of brown and white rice flour for your breads.

Stir in any additional ingredients called for in a recipe such as fruit, raisins, or nuts just before putting the dough in the pans. If there is a special seasoning such as spices or herbs, these are added to the dry ingredients.

BASIC FORMULA FOR MAKING BREAD BY HAND

Have all the ingredients at room temperature except the liquid, which should test about 110°.

Mix the dry ingredients and, in most cases, add the yeast granules to the flour mix.

In the bowl of a heavy-duty mixer, beat the eggs with the dough enhancer or vinegar until foamy. Add the other liquid ingredients including most of the warm water, holding back several tablespoons to add later, if needed.

With the beater on low, spoon in the dry ingredients slowly. If you don't, you'll have flour all over the kitchen. Check to see if the batter is the right texture. It should look much like cake batter. If it seems too thick, add water a tablespoonful at a time until you are satisfied with the texture, but don't thin too much since the beating that follows will thin it some. Turn the beater to high and mix for about 3½ minutes. Spoon the dough into the pan (or pans) that have been greased and dusted with rice flour.

Cover with a light cloth or paper toweling and set aside in a draft-free place to rise. Preheat the oven to the recipe's suggested temperature. When the dough has almost doubled in bulk (about 35 to 45 minutes for rapid-rising yeast and double that time for regular), place the pans in the oven, leaving space around them.

After the first 10 minutes of baking, cover with aluminum foil. To test for doneness, thump the bread before removing from the oven. It should sound hollow, and the crust should not be so tender that your finger can dent it easily. Tip out of the pans immediately after removing them from the oven. If you want a more tender crust, rub with margarine while still hot.

BUYING AND USING A BREAD MACHINE

With the coming of the bread machines a few years ago, the problem of making our bread seemed to be solved. We could just dump in the ingredients and let the machine do the work, couldn't we? It's not quite that simple for not all machines are suited to making our heavy breads.

When they first came out, I tested many machines, but in the last few years the overwhelming number on the market made this impossible. But if you decide to invest in one, there are certain features you should look for.

1. A heavy-duty motor and large paddle (or paddles). The dough-hook-shaped paddle is not best for our dough. Some machines have a short thick paddle, and this, too, will work only if the dough is mixed outside the pan or you use a rubber spatula to stir the dough as it is mixing.
2. A cycle that can be programmed to cut out the "stir down" or second rising. Our dough does not take well to this process since the yeast is not feeding on gluten as it would in wheat flours. If the machine cannot be programmed to avoid the stir down, check to see whether it is possible to remove the paddles after the first mixing to avoid rebeating the dough.
3. A program that lets you switch manually from Kneading to Rising to Bake, thus controlling all the cycles for the best rising and baking. Using this will mean that you have to stand over the machine and watch the bread as it proofs.
4. A cool-down cycle so the bread doesn't stand in the pan and turn soggy if you don't remove it immediately. This is not as important as the other features if you are planning to stay nearby during the baking.
5. Two paddles rather than a single one in the center if the machine has an oblong, loaf-shaped pan. Otherwise you'll have to continually stir the corners during the kneading process.

Since companies are constantly changing their machines and new companies are entering the field, it would be wise to get recommendations from others who are baking with gluten-free flour. Ask what they like and what they would change about their machines.

Yeast Breads

True Yeast Bread (Revised) 400°

When gluten intolerance was first recognized, there were no recipes for a yeast bread without wheat. This formula, adapted from one created in the nutrition department of the University of Washington School of Medicine, was one of the first developed at the time this book was published. Since then I've updated and revised it.

3 cups GF Mix or Four Flour Bean Mix (pages 38–39)
¼ cup sugar
2½ teaspoons xanthan gum
½ cup dry milk powder or nondairy substitute
1 teaspoon unflavored gelatin
1½ teaspoons Egg Replacer
¾ teaspoon salt
2 teaspoons sugar
½ cup lukewarm water (110°)
1 tablespoon yeast granules
¼ cup shortening
1¼ cups water (more or less)
1 teaspoon vinegar or dough enhancer
1 egg plus 2 egg whites

Grease an 8½″ × 4½″ loaf pan plus 6 muffin cups or 3 small 2½″ × 5″ loaf pans and dust with rice flour.

For hand mixing: In the bowl of a heavy-duty mixer, combine flour mix, ¼ cup sugar, xanthan gum, milk powder, unflavored gelatin, Egg Replacer, and salt. Use the flat beater, not the dough hook.

Dissolve the 2 teaspoons sugar in the lukewarm water and mix in the yeast. Set aside. Combine the shortening and water in a saucepan and heat until shortening melts.

Turn mixer on low. Blend dry ingredients and slowly add shortening and water mixture and vinegar. Blend, then add egg and egg whites. This mixture should feel slightly warm. Pour in the yeast water and beat at highest speed for 3½ minutes. The texture of the dough will be more like cake batter than regular bread dough, so don't be alarmed.

Spoon the dough into the prepared pans. Let rise until doubled in bulk (35 to 45 minutes for rapid-rising yeast; 60 to 70 minutes for regular). Bake in a preheated 400° oven for 50 minutes for the larger loaf, slightly less for the small loaves, and 25 minutes for the rolls, covering after the first 10 minutes with aluminum foil.

For bread machine: Combine the dry ingredients as for hand mixing but add the yeast to the flours. In another bowl, blend all the wet ingredients. Place them in the machine following instructions in your machine's manual.

Nutrients per serving: Calories 130, Fat 4 g, Carbohydrate 20 g, Cholesterol 30 mg, Sodium 160 mg, Fiber 0, Protein 3 g

GRANOLA BREAD: Add ¼ cup granola to the dry ingredients.

SEED AND NUT BREAD: Add 2 tablespoons either chopped pumpkin or sunflower seeds plus 2 tablespoons chopped nuts to the dry ingredients.

CINNAMON-RAISIN-NUT BREAD: Add ¾ teaspoon cinnamon to the dry ingredients and stir in 2 tablespoons raisins and 2 tablespoons chopped nuts before spooning into pans.

Hamburger Buns

375°

Follow the recipe above for True Yeast Bread but shape some or all as follows:

Use eight 4-inch English muffin rings as forms. Grease them inside and place on well-greased cookie sheet. Or make your own forms for containing the dough by taking a sheet of foil (about 10 inches torn from roll), folding it in half, then half again and again until you get a strong strip slightly over 1 inch wide. Tape the ends together with masking tape to form a circle. Grease the inside, and place on greased cookie sheets. Spoon your bread dough into these forms, filling only half full.

Let rise to double in height and bake in a preheated 375° oven for 20 to 25 minutes. *Makes 8 buns.*

Nutrients per serving: Calories 390, Fat 12 g, Carbohydrate 60 g, Cholesterol 90 mg, Sodium 480 mg, Fiber 0, Protein 9 g

Four Flour Bread 400°

This is a mild-flavored basic bread that can take any kind of additions including grains, nuts, seeds, spices, and even other flours. Make it with water, as the recipe suggests, or use fruit juice, milk (or nondairy substitute), or a carbonated beverage. Use your imagination or get ideas from the many bread recipes now being published for wheat breads. This recipe may be doubled for 2 loaves or a two-pound bread machine. Do not double the yeast.

2 cups Four Flour Bean Mix
1½ teaspoons xanthan gum
½ teaspoon salt
1 teaspoon unflavored gelatin
1 teaspoon Egg Replacer
2 tablespoons sugar
2¼ teaspoons dry yeast granules
1 egg plus 1 egg white
3 tablespoons margarine or butter
1 teaspoon dough enhancer or vinegar
1 cup (more or less) warm water

Grease an 8½" × 4½" loaf pan and dust with rice flour or plan to use a 1-pound bread machine.

The water temperature will be different for hand mixing and bread machines. For hand mixing have it about 110° to 115°. For your bread machine, refer to the directions in the manual.

For both hand mixing and machine mixing, combine the flour mix, xanthan gum, salt, gelatin, Egg Replacer, sugar, and yeast in a medium bowl. Set aside.

In another bowl (or the bowl of a heavy-duty mixer), whisk the egg and egg white, margarine, and dough enhancer. Add most of the water. The remaining water should be added as needed after the bread has started mixing, in the bowl of the mixer or in the pan of the bread machine.

For hand mixing: With the mixer turned low, add the flour mix (including the yeast) a little at a time. Check to be sure the dough is the right consistency (should be like cake batter). Add more of the reserved water as necessary. Turn mixer to high and beat for 3½ minutes. Spoon dough into prepared pan, cover, and let rise in a warm place about 35 to 45 minutes for rapid-rising yeast, 60 or more minutes for regular yeast (or until the dough reaches the top of the pan). Bake in a preheated 400° oven for 50 to 60 minutes, covering after 10 minutes with aluminum foil.

For bread machine: Place wet and dry ingredients in bread machine in the order suggested by machine manual. Use the setting for white bread with medium crust.

LEMON–POPPY SEED BREAD: Add 2 teaspoons dried lemon peel and 2 teaspoons poppy seeds to the dry ingredients.

QUINOA BREAD: Add 2 tablespoons quinoa flour to the dry ingredients; add 2 teaspoons honey to the wet ingredients.

ALMOND BREAD: Add 3 tablespoons almond meal to the dry ingredients; add 1 teaspoon almond flavor to the wet ingredients.

CINNAMON-NUT BREAD: Add 1 teaspoon cinnamon to the dry ingredients. Stir in ¼ cup chopped nuts after the dough is mixed when baking by hand or when manual suggests when using machine.

SESAME BEAN BREAD: Add 2 tablespoons toasted sesame seeds to the dry ingredients; 2 teaspoons molasses to the wet ingredients.

Nutrients per slice: Calories 130, Fat 4 g, Carbohydrate 29 g,
Cholesterol 25 mg, Sodium 150 mg, Fiber 9 g, Protein 3 g

Sticky Pecan Rolls 375°

Follow the recipe for True Yeast Bread but instead of putting in pans, place about 2 cups of dough on buttered wax paper. With well-greased hands pat it out to about ⅓ inch thick in a rectangular shape. Then:

Spread with a mixture of ¼ cup (½ stick) softened butter and ¼ cup brown sugar.
Sprinkle on ½ cup chopped pecans

Form a roll, carefully working the sticky dough from the waxed paper. Don't worry if it doesn't become smooth or look perfect.

Seal the roll and then slice in about 1¼-inch pieces. Put pieces in muffin tins greased with an extra dab of butter on the bottom and let rise until doubled in bulk.

Bake in a preheated 375° oven for 20 minutes.

Nutrients per roll: Calories 180, Fat 9 g, Carbohydrate 24 g, Cholesterol 35 mg, Sodium 210 mg, Fiber 1 g, Protein 3 g

Easy Cinnamon-Nut Rolls 400°

These are much easier than the Sticky Pecan Rolls above and turn out deliciously sticky and sweet!

1 recipe True Yeast Bread (page 53) or 1½ recipes Four Flour Bean Bread (38–39) (increase sugar to ½ cup)
4 tablespoons margarine or butter
⅓ cup chopped pecans or walnuts
⅓ cup brown sugar
1 teaspoon cinnamon
⅓ cup raisins
½ teaspoon dried orange peel

Lightly grease 18 muffin cups. Divide the margarine among the 18 cups, placing about 1 teaspoon in each.

In a medium bowl, blend the nuts, brown sugar, cinnamon, raisins, and dried orange peel.

Fill the muffin tins by alternating the nut mixture and bread dough. Start with ½ teaspoon of the nut mixture, then 1 heaping tablespoon of dough, another nut mixture, another dough. Top with the nut mixture.

Cover and let rise for 25 to 30 minutes. Bake in a preheated 400° oven for 20 to 25 minutes. Serve warm or cold. *Makes 18 rolls.*

Nutrients per roll: Calories 110, Fat 5 g, Carbohydrate 16 g, Cholesterol 20 mg, Sodium 115 mg, Fiber 0, Protein 2 g

Sourdough Bread

If you miss the sourdough breads of "before diagnosis days," try this new and springy version made with either bean or rice flour. Since sourdough begins with a starter, we celiacs can't buy one, so have to make our own. This is made, fermented, and then replenished each time it is used. The older the starter, the more taste the bread will have.

If you are making new starter, it should be made at least one day before you plan to bake. Three days is better. Store it in its crock or glass jar (never metal or plastic) on the kitchen counter or in the refrigerator. If refrigerated, take it out at least 10 hours before baking, or the night before.

Rice flour works well for a starter for both rice- and bean-based breads.

Starter

2¼ teaspoons dry yeast granules
1 cup lukewarm potato water or water with 1 teaspoon instant potato flakes
1 teaspoon sugar
1 cup white rice flour

In a 1- or 1½-quart glass jar or pottery crock, dissolve the yeast in the potato water. Stir in the sugar and rice flour. Cover and let the jar sit out until fermented (1 to 3 days), stirring every few hours at first. This will bubble up and ferment and then die down with a skim of liquid on the top. Be sure to stir well before using. The consistency should be about that of pancake batter.

Replenish after use by feeding the remaining starter with ½ cup (or 1 cup) lukewarm water and ¾ cup (or 1½ cups) rice flour, as needed, each time you bake.

Buttermilk Sourdough 400°

This light and springy sourdough can be made with either bean or rice flour. The rice will not rise as high as the bean flour loaf, but the texture will be fine with no crumbling. Try the rye variation listed below for variety. The recipe may be doubled for two loaves or a large bread machine.

Note: The amount of yeast is cut when sourdough starter is used. If baking in the oven, you may increase the yeast slightly for a quicker rise, but don't attempt this if using a bread machine.

2 cups Fours Flour Bean Mix or GF Mix (pages 38–39)
1½ teaspoons xanthan gum
½ teaspoon salt
1 teaspoon Egg Replacer
1 teaspoon unflavored gelatin
⅓ cup buttermilk powder
1 teaspoon dried lemon peel
3 tablespoons sugar
1½ teaspoons dry yeast granules
1 egg plus 1 egg white
½ teaspoon dough enhancer or vinegar
½ cup sourdough starter
3 tablespoons vegetable oil
1 cup (more or less) warm water

Grease an 8½″ × 4½″ loaf pan and dust with rice flour or set bread machine to program white bread with medium crust.

The water temperature will be different for hand mixing and for different brands of bread machines. For hand mixing have it about 110°. For your bread machine, refer to the manual directions.

For both hand mixing and machine mixing, in a medium bowl combine the flour mix, xanthan gum, salt, Egg Replacer, gelatin, buttermilk powder, lemon peel, and sugar. Set aside.

In another bowl (or the bowl of a heavy-duty mixer), whisk the egg and egg white, dough enhancer, sourdough starter, vegetable oil, and most of the water. The remaining water should be added as needed after the bread has started mixing either in the bowl of the heavy-duty mixer or in the pan of the bread machine.

For hand mixing: With the mixer turned low, add the flour mix (including the yeast) a little at a time. Check to be sure the dough is thin enough (like a thick cake batter for the rice flour and a little thinner for the bean flour). Add more of the reserved water as necessary. Turn mixer to high and beat for 3½ minutes. Spoon the dough into the prepared pan, cover, and let rise about 35 to 45 minutes for rapid-rising yeast; 60 or more minutes for regular yeast (or until the bread has risen about half more than its original size). Note: This is not the same as most dough, which almost doubles in bulk. Bake in a preheated 400° oven for 55 to 60 minutes, covering after 10 minutes with aluminum foil.

For bread machine: Place in bread machine pan in the order suggested by your machine manual.

Nutrients per slice: Calories 160, Fat 3 g, Carbohydrate 29 g, Cholesterol 35 mg, Sodium 150 mg, Fiber 1 g, Protein 5 g

BUTTERMILK SOURDOUGH RYE: To the dry ingredients add 1 teaspoon caraway seeds, 1 teaspoon cardamom, and ⅛ teaspoon rye flavor powder (which may be ordered from Authentic Foods). Substitute brown sugar for the sugar.

Tapioca Bread

400°

For a fine, white, springy-textured bread try this rice and tapioca flour mixture. You will find it tastes like wheat flour breads.

2 cups rice flour
1½ cups tapioca flour
¼ cup sugar
2½ teaspoons xanthan gum
½ cup dry milk powder or nondairy substitute
¾ teaspoon salt
1 tablespoon dry yeast granules
½ cup lukewarm water
2 teaspoons sugar
¼ cup shortening
1¼ cups hot water
1 teaspoon vinegar or dough enhancer
1 egg plus 2 egg whites or ¾ cup liquid egg substitute

Grease two 8½″ × 4½″ loaf pans and dust with rice flour.

Combine flours, sugar, xanthan gum, milk powder, and salt in the large bowl of a heavy-duty mixer. In a separate bowl, sprinkle yeast into the lukewarm water with the 2 teaspoons of sugar added, and let dissolve. Melt shortening in 1¼ cups of water.

Pour shortening mixture and vinegar into dry ingredients and blend on low. Add egg and egg whites and beat a few seconds. Add the dissolved yeast. Beat at highest speed for 3½ minutes.

Spoon dough into prepared pans. Let dough rise until doubled in bulk (35 to 40 minutes for rapid-rising yeast, 60 to 75 minutes for regular).

Bake in a preheated 400° oven for 50 to 60 minutes. Cover after the first 10 minutes with aluminum foil.

Nutrients per serving: Calories 130, Fat 4 g, Carbohydrate 29 g, Cholesterol 30 mg, Sodium 170 mg, Fiber 10 g, Protein 3 g

Easy French Bread

400°, 350°

If you're craving that crusty-outside, soft-inside French bread taste, try this mix that has little sugar and only a trace of fat. This is so good, your friends won't believe it is gluten free. This bread is especially sensitive to humidity and works best at times of low humidity. Damp weather tends to make the bread soggy.

¾ cup white rice flour
⅔ cup cornstarch
⅔ cup tapioca flour
2 teaspoons potato flour
2½ teaspoons xanthan gum
2 teaspoons Egg Replacer
1 teaspoon salt
2 teaspoons unflavored gelatin
⅓ cup dry milk powder or nondairy substitute
1 tablespoon sugar
1¼ cups warm water (110°)
1 tablespoon dry yeast granules
1 teaspoon dough enhancer or vinegar
2 egg whites
1½ tablespoons vegetable oil

Grease two 14″ French loaf pans or one cookie sheet. Dust with cornmeal (if desired).

In the bowl of your heavy-duty mixer, place the rice flour, cornstarch, tapioca flour, potato flour, xanthan gum, Egg Replacer, salt, unflavored gelatin, and milk powder.

Place the sugar in the warm water and stir in the yeast. Set aside to foam.

Add to the dry ingredients in the mixing bowl the dough enhancer, egg whites, and vegetable oil. When the foam on the yeast is about ½ inch, pour this into the dry mix. Beat on high for 3 minutes. Spoon into the prepared loaf pans or onto the prepared cookie sheet in two French bread loaf shapes. Brush lightly with wet fingers to smooth the tops and then slash diagonally every few inches. Cover the loaves and let rise in a warm place until almost doubled (about 35 minutes for rapid-rising yeast; 1 hour for regular yeast).

Bake in a preheated 400° oven for 15 minutes. Then turn oven to 350° and bake 30 minutes more. *Makes two 10-inch loaves.*

Nutrients per serving: Calories 70, Fat 1.5 g, Carbohydrate 12 g, Cholesterol 0, Sodium 105 mg, Fiber 0, Protein 2 g

Bread Sticks

400°

Instead of forming loaves, use the French bread recipe above and spoon the dough into a plastic freezer bag with ½ inch of one corner cut off. Squeeze the dough in strips onto 2 greased cookie sheets. The recipe will make about a dozen 12-inch sticks or two dozen 6-inch sticks.

Let rise until doubled in size and bake about 20–25 minutes in preheated 400° oven. Serving size: one 12-inch stick or two 6-inch sticks.

Nutrients per serving: Calories 105, Fat 2.3 g, Carbohydrate 18 g, Cholesterol 0, Sodium 157 mg, Fiber 0, Protein 3 g

Steve's Cheesy Bread Sticks

400°

A fellow celiac brought these to one of our picnics. They were so delicious I begged for the recipe. Try these soft and chewy bread sticks for a snack, with soups, or when traveling.

⅓ cup Garfava flour
½ cup white rice flour
⅔ cup tapioca flour
½ cup cornstarch
⅓ cup dry milk powder or nondairy substitute
1½ teaspoons xanthan gum
½ teaspoon salt
1 tablespoon dry yeast granules
½ cup warm water (110°)
2 teaspoons sugar
1½ tablespoons margarine or butter
¼ cup hot water
2 egg whites
1 cup grated sharp Cheddar cheese

Preheat oven to 400°. Grease a cookie sheet. Cut an opening 1 inch across the corner of a strong plastic storage bag.

In bowl of mixer, place flours, cornstarch, milk powder, xanthan gum, and salt. Blend on low.

Dissolve the sugar in the warm water and sprinkle in the yeast. Let this foam.

Put butter to melt in the hot water.

Add butter-water mixture to dry ingredients and blend. Add the egg whites and blend. Pour in yeast mixture and beat on high for 4 minutes. Stir in the cheese. The dough should be thick but still thin enough to easily press through the opening of the plastic bag. If too thick, thin with warm water, adding only 1 teaspoon at a time.

Press out in five 14-inch-long strips down the length of the cookie sheet. Let rise 20 minutes and then bake for 18 to 20 minutes or until golden brown on top. Remove to a rack to cool. Cut into 2½-inch sections. *Makes 25 servings.*

Nutrients per serving: Calories 160, Fat 12 g, Carbohydrate 10 g, Cholesterol 5 mg, Sodium 210 mg, Fiber 0, Protein 3 g

Challah

400°

(a lactose-free, soy-free bread)

A boon for those who are both lactose and soy intolerant and cannot use the soy-based nondairy substitutes for the dry powdered milk in the other bread recipes. This is an excellent-tasting bread with a rich flavor, so it can be eaten with just butter or in any kind of sandwich.

1½ tablespoons sesame seeds
2 cups rice flour
1¾ cups tapioca flour
¼ cup sugar
3 teaspoons xanthan gum
2 teaspoons unflavored gelatin
1 teaspoon salt
1 tablespoon dry yeast granules
½ cup lukewarm water
2 teaspoons sugar
¼ cup shortening
1¼ cups hot water
1 teaspoon vinegar or dough enhancer
3 eggs, at room temperature
2 egg yolks

Grease two 8½″ × 4½″ loaf pans and dust with rice flour.

Brown sesame seeds in heavy skillet on medium heat. Set aside. Combine flours, sugar, xanthan gum, gelatin, and salt in bowl of mixer. Blend. In a separate bowl, dissolve yeast in warm water to which the 2 teaspoons of sugar have been added. Soften the shortening in the hot water.

Pour shortening mixture into dry ingredients, add vinegar, and blend on low. Add eggs and egg yolks, beating slightly. The mixture should be slightly warm. Add yeast water and beat 3½ minutes on high. Stir in most of the toasted sesame seeds, reserving a pinch or two for the top.

Spoon dough into prepared pans. Sprinkle with the remaining sesame seeds. Let dough rise again in a warm place until doubled, approximately 35 to 45 minutes for rapid-rising yeast; 60 to 70 minutes for regular.

Bake in a preheated 400° oven for 50 to 60 minutes, covering after the first 10 minutes with aluminum foil.

This bread freezes well. Cool and slice before freezing.

Nutrients per slice: Calories 160, Fat 4 g, Carbohydrate 28 g, Cholesterol 45 mg, Sodium 150 mg, Fiber 1 g, Protein 3 g

Single-Rising Coffee Bread — 375°

An easy-to-make, fine-grained sweet yeast bread that is good with just butter or with jam. This bread will take the addition of raisins, spices, or nuts for an entirely different taste. The use of both baking powder and yeast as leavening agents gives it an unusual flavor.

2 cups GF Mix or Four Flour Bean Mix (pages 38–39)
4 teaspoons baking powder
¼ cup sugar
¼ cup powdered milk or nondairy substitute
½ teaspoon salt
1½ teaspoons xanthan gum
1 teaspoon unflavored gelatin
1 teaspoon Egg Replacer
½ cup shortening
1 tablespoon dry yeast granules
¾ cup warm water
1 tablespoon sugar
2 eggs, at room temperature

Place flour, baking powder, sugar, dry milk, salt, xanthan gum, unflavored gelatin, and Egg Replacer in large bowl of mixer. Cut in the shortening. In a separate bowl, dissolve yeast in warm water to which 1 tablespoon of sugar has been added. Add with the eggs to the flour mixture. Beat 5 minutes. The dough will be very thick.

Grease hands and knead dough using a rice-floured board. Pat into round shape about 8 inches in diameter and approximately 2 inches thick at center.

Let stand 40 minutes or more until doubled in size.

Bake on a greased cookie sheet in a preheated 375° oven for 40 minutes covered with aluminum foil to prevent dark crust.

NOTE: Those who are both lactose and soy intolerant can eliminate the powdered milk and replace the water and powdered milk with ¾ cup fruit juice (orange, pear, or other). Add 2 extra egg whites for protein. Remember to add the extra tablespoon of sugar to the juice to help the yeast work.

JULEKAKA: Turn the above bread into a Christmas loaf by adding 1 teaspoon dried orange rind and 1 cup chopped candied fruit. (A yeast-free Christmas bread can be found on page 199.)

CINNAMON-NUT BREAD: Another variation can be made by adding 1 teaspoon cinnamon to the flours and stirring in ½ to 1 cup chopped nuts at the end of the beating.

Nutrients per slice: Calories 140, Fat 7 g, Carbohydrate 19 g, Cholesterol 25 mg, Sodium 467 mg, Fiber 0, Protein 2 g

Dilly Casserole Bread 350°

This is an unusual and excitingly flavored bread made in a round shape and baked in a casserole. It is wonderful with just butter and makes a fine accompaniment to soups. It also makes a hearty sandwich with strong-tasting fillings like ham, cheese, or corned beef.

1 packet dry yeast granules
¼ cup warm water
2 tablespoons sugar
1 cup creamed cottage cheese
2 eggs, at room temperature
2 teaspoons dill seed
½ teaspoon salt
½ teaspoon baking soda
1 tablespoon butter or margarine
1 tablespoon instant minced onion
2 cups GF Mix or Four Flour Bean Mix (pages 38–39)
1½ teaspoons xanthan gum
1 teaspoon Egg Replacer

Soften yeast in the warm water to which the sugar has been added. Warm cottage cheese to lukewarm.

Combine in bowl of mixer all the ingredients except the flours, xanthan gum, and Egg Replacer. Combine the flours, xanthan gum, and Egg Replacer and add slowly, beating after each addition, until you have a stiff dough.

Let rise until doubled in bulk (35 to 40 minutes for rapid-rising yeast; 60 to 75 minutes for regular). Bake in a preheated 350° oven for 40 to 50 minutes, until golden. Brush with soft butter.

Nutrients per slice: Calories 110, Fat 2 g, Carbohydrate 18 g, Cholesterol 30 mg, Sodium 160 mg, Fiber 1 g, Protein 3 g

Almost Pumpernickel 400°

You won't believe this isn't the real thing! This is great for sandwiches with strong meats like ham and corned beef or your favorite cheese. Use it on the buffet table cut into quarters and topped with the Ham and Cheese Spread (page 255). Cut a slice into triangles and toast it to serve with cavier—if you can afford it after buying your gluten-free foods.

This recipe may be doubled for two loaves or for a 2-pound bread machine but do not double the yeast.

- 2 cups Four Flour Bean Mix or GF Mix (pages 38–39)
- 1½ teaspoons xanthan gum
- ½ teaspoon salt
- 1 teaspoon unflavored gelatin
- 1 teaspoon Egg Replacer
- 2 tablespoons brown sugar
- 2 tablespoons dry milk powder or nondairy substitute (optional)
- 2 teaspoons cocoa powder
- 2 teaspoons caraway seeds
- 2¼ teaspoons dry yeast granules
- 1 egg plus 1 egg white
- 2 tablespoons vegetable oil
- 1 teaspoon dough enhancer or vinegar
- 2 tablespoons molasses
- 1 cup warm water (more or less)

Grease an 8½″ × 4½″ loaf pan and dust with rice flour or use the 1 # bread machine.

The water temperature will be different for hand mixing and bread machines. For hand mixing have it about 110°; for the bread machine follow the directions in the manual.

For both hand mixing and machine mixing, combine the flour mix, xanthan gum, salt, gelatin, Egg Replacer, brown sugar, milk powder (if used), cocoa powder, caraway seeds, and yeast. Set aside.

In another bowl (or the bowl of a heavy-duty mixer), whisk the egg and egg white slightly; add vegetable oil, dough enchancer, molasses, and most of the water. The remaining water should be added as needed after the bread has started mixing, either in bowl of mixer or in pan of bread machine.

For hand mixing: With the mixer turned to low, add dry ingredients (including yeast) a little at a time. Be sure dough is the right consistency (like cake batter). Add more water if necessary. Turn mixer to high and beat for 3½ minutes. Spoon dough into prepared pan, cover, and let rise about 35 to 45 minutes for rapid-rising yeast, 60 or more minutes for regular yeast, or until dough has reached top of pan. Bake in a preheated 400° oven for 50 to 60 minutes, covering after 10 minutes with aluminum foil.

For bread machine: Place ingredients in bread machine in the order suggested in the machine manual. Use setting for white bread with medium crust.

Nutrients per slice: Calories 140, Fat 4 g, Carbohydrate 24 g, Cholesterol 20 mg, Sodium 120 mg, Fiber 1 g, Protein 4 g

Cheese Bread 400°

A good introduction to bean flour in a rice bread with a touch of bean. This is easy to beat up in one bowl in your mixer. And the flavor is delicious. See the variations for other tastes. This recipe makes one loaf. It may be doubled for two loaves.

⅓ cup Garfava flour
½ cup white rice flour
⅔ cup tapioca flour
½ cup cornstarch
1½ teaspoons xanthan gum
1 teaspoon Egg Replacer
1 teaspoon unflavored gelatin
⅓ cup dry milk powder or nondairy substitute
½ teaspoon salt
2 teaspoons sugar
½ cup warm water (110°–115°)
1 tablespoon dry yeast granules
2 tablespoons butter or margarine
½ cup hot water
2 egg whites
1 cup grated sharp Cheddar cheese

Grease an 8½″ × 4½″ loaf pan and dust with rice flour.

In bowl of heavy-duty mixer, place Garfava flour, rice flour, tapioca flour, cornstarch, xanthan gum, Egg Replacer, gelatin, milk powder, and salt. Blend on low.

Dissolve sugar in warm water and sprinkle in yeast. Let this foam.

Put butter to melt in hot water.

Add most of butter-water mixture to dry ingredients and blend. (Hold back some to add later if needed.) Add egg whites and blend. Pour in yeast mixture and blend. Check to see if dough is the consistency of thick cake batter. Add more reserved water as needed. Beat on high for 4 minutes. Stir in cheese.

Spoon into prepared pan, cover, and let rise until almost doubled in bulk or until it reaches top of pan (35 to 45 minutes for rapid-rising yeast, 50 to 65 minutes for regular yeast). Bake in a preheated 400° oven for 50 to 60 minutes, covering after the first 10 minutes with aluminum foil to prevent overbrowning. *Makes 1 loaf.*

CHEESE-ONION BREAD: Add 1 tablespoon dry minced onion.

PIZZA BREAD: Add 2 teaspoons Pizza Seasoning (or to taste).

Nutrients per slice: Calories 140, Fat 6 g, Carbohydrate 16 g, Cholesterol 20 mg, Sodium 190 mg, Fiber 1 g, Protein 6 g

Quick-Rising Breads

Yeast-free Bean-Sorghum Bread 350°

You won't believe this isn't a yeast bread. For those who can't have yeast, this is a bread to live with. Use it plain or make one of the variations listed below. This recipe may be doubled to make two loaves. Not suitable for bread machines.

2 cups Four-Flour Bean Mix (pages 38–39)
1½ teaspoons xanthan gum
3 tablespoons brown sugar
½ teaspoon baking soda
2 teaspoons baking powder
1 teaspoon Egg Replacer
½ teaspoon salt
2 eggs plus 1 egg white
3 tablespoons margarine or butter, melted
1 tablespoon honey
½ teaspoon dough enhancer (optional)
¾ cup buttermilk
¼ cup water (more or less)

Preheat oven to 350°. Grease an 8½″ × 4½″ loaf pan and dust with rice flour.

In a medium bowl, whisk together the flour mix, xanthan gum, brown sugar, baking soda, baking powder, Egg Replacer, and salt. Set aside.

In the bowl of your mixer, beat eggs and egg white. Add the melted margarine, honey, dough enhancer (if used), and buttermilk. Turn mixer to low and blend. Add the dry ingredients while on low. Add sufficient water to make dough the consistency of cake batter. Beat 1 minute on high. Spoon into prepared pan and bake for 55 to 60 minutes, covering after 30 minutes with aluminum foil.

POPPY SEED LOAF: Eliminate honey from wet ingredients and add 2 teaspoons poppy seeds and 1 teaspoon dried lemon peel to dry ingredients.

CINNAMON-RAISIN-NUT LOAF: Add ½ teaspoon cinnamon to dry ingredients, and after beating, stir in 3 tablespoons each chopped nuts and raisins.

SESAME SEED LOAF: Add 2 teaspoons sesame seeds to dry ingredients and substitute molasses for the honey in wet ingredients.

Nutrients per slice: Calories 100, Fat 3 g, Carbohydrate 16 g,
Cholesterol 25 mg, Sodium 110 mg, Fiber 1 g, Protein 2 g

Potato-Rice Sponge Bread 350°

This is a fine eating bread with jam or spreads. It is good toasted or used for french toast. Since it contains no yeast, it is a good substitute if you cannot tolerate yeast products.

6 eggs, at room temperature
2½ tablespoons sugar
¾ cup potato starch flour
½ cup rice flour
1 teaspoon salt
2 teaspoons baking powder
2 teaspoons Egg Replacer (optional)

Separate eggs. In large bowl, beat egg whites until mounds form. Then beat in the sugar a tablespoon at a time. In another bowl, beat egg yolks until light, creamy, and fluffy, approximately 5 minutes at high speed.

Sift together the flours, salt, baking powder, and Egg Replacer. Sprinkle about one-third of the flour mixture over the whites; fold together gently until well mixed; repeat two times. Carefully fold beaten egg yolks into flour mixture until well blended.

Pour batter into coated nonstick 8½″ × 4½″ × 3″ loaf pan. Bake in a preheated 350° oven for 45 to 50 minutes. Cool 1 hour before removing from pan. Allow to cool 3 hours before slicing.

Nutrients per slice: Calories 80, Fat 2 g, Carbohydrate 12 g, Cholesterol 80 mg, Sodium 210 mg, Fiber 0, Protein 3 g

Best Banana Bread 350°

After trying many banana breads that crumbled on cutting, I discovered a combination of flours, including soy, that turns out a firm loaf. The texture is fine and the flavor is nutty banana without being too sweet. You may replace the three flours with 1¾ cups Four Flour Bean Mix (pages 38–39*).*

1 cup soy flour
½ cup potato starch flour
¼ cup rice flour
½ teaspoon xanthan gum
1 teaspoon baking soda
1¼ teaspoons cream of tartar
½ teaspoon salt
⅓ cup shortening
⅔ cup sugar
2 eggs, well beaten
½ cup mashed banana
½ cup chopped nuts (optional)

Preheat oven to 350°. Grease an 8½″ × 4½″ loaf pan.

In a medium bowl, whisk together the flours, xanthan gum, baking soda, cream of tartar, and salt. Set aside.

In a mixing bowl, cream shortening. Gradually add the sugar, beating until light and fluffy. Add the well-beaten eggs. Beat well. Add the dry ingredients alternately with the mashed banana, a small amount at a time, beating after each addition until smooth.

Stir in the chopped nuts (if used). Pour into prepared pan and bake for 1 hour.

Nutrients per slice: Calories 220, Fat 10 g, Carbohydrate 29 g, Cholesterol 35 mg, Sodium 180 mg, Fiber 1 g, Protein 4 g

Hawaiian Tea Bread 350°

This "party" bread with a hint of sunny tropical isles can be served in place of cake. And it can be served not only to those with gluten and lactose intolerance but, with a slight change in recipe, to those who can't have eggs. But hide some to save for yourself.

⅓ cup (⅔ stick) margarine, softened
⅔ cup honey
2 eggs, beaten, or ¼ cup vegetable oil
2 tablespoons water
½ teaspoon vanilla
1 cup rice flour
½ cup rice polish
1 teaspoon baking powder
½ teaspoon baking soda
½ teaspoon xanthan gum
1 cup grated coconut, sweetened or unsweetened
1 cup chopped walnuts (optional)
4 ripe bananas, sliced thin

In a large mixing bowl, cream margarine. Beat while adding honey in a fine stream. Beat in eggs, or oil if you are allergic to eggs. Stir in water and vanilla. In a separate bowl, sift together rice flour, rice polish, baking powder, baking soda, and xanthan gum. Add coconut and walnuts (if used).

Add dry ingredients alternately with bananas to the creamed mixture, folding only until everything is moistened. Spoon into greased 9″ × 5″ loaf pan. Bake for 55 minutes in preheated 350° oven. Allow to cool in pan for 5 minutes before removing.

Nutrients per slice: Calories 220, Fat 10 g, Carbohydrate 31 g, Cholesterol 25 mg, Sodium 85 mg, Fiber 1 g, Protein 3 g

Apricot Bread

350°

A different fruit-flavored bread for those who are tired of banana. The texture of this is slightly grainier than that of the banana bread, but the flavor more than compensates. It is good plain as a coffee cake, with just butter, or, for a lunch-box treat, serve with cream cheese or other mild-tasting cheese.

If you prefer, you may eliminate the soy flour and use 2 cups of rice flour. I like the taste with the soy added, but the recipe will turn out well either way.

1 cup apricot purée
½ cup sugar
2 tablespoons shortening
2 eggs
1½ cups rice flour
½ cup soy flour
½ teaspoon xanthan gum
1 tablespoon baking powder
½ teaspoon baking soda
1 teaspoon salt
1 tablespoon grated orange peel
½ cup orange juice
1 cup chopped nuts

Preheat oven to 350°. Grease a 9″ × 5″ loaf pan.

Purée apricots in blender. Set aside. (Use canned apricots, drained, or dried apricots, cooked and drained.)

Cream sugar and shortening. Add eggs and puréed apricots. Mix well. Sift the flours, xanthan gum, baking powder, baking soda, and salt. Add orange peel.

Add flour mixture alternately with the orange juice to the creamed mixture. Beat lightly and stir in the nuts.

Pour into prepared pan and bake until the bread pulls away from the sides and is lightly browned, approximately 45 to 50 minutes.

The bread is better if ripened overnight before serving.

If desired, the bread may be divided into two 4″ × 8″ pans. The cooking time will be shorter.

Nutrients per slice: Calories 210, Fat 7 g, Carbohydrate 34 g, Cholesterol 35 mg, Sodium 340 mg, Fiber 1 g, Protein 4 g

Pumpkin Bread 350°

One of the best of the sweet breads. The texture of this rivals any bread made with gluten flour. It stays moist and doesn't need heating to taste good. The spices, pumpkin, and pecans give it a flavor reminiscent of pumpkin pie. But don't save this just for Thanksgiving. It is good anytime.

1 cup GF Mix (page 38)
½ teaspoon xanthan gum
½ teaspoon baking soda
1½ teaspoons baking powder
¼ cup sugar
½ teaspoon salt
1½ teaspoons pumpkin pie spice
2 eggs
⅔ cup canned pumpkin
¼ cup mayonnaise
2 tablespoons chopped pecans, or 2 tablespoons chopped dates or raisins

Preheat oven to 350°. Grease an 8½″ × 4½″ loaf pan or two 5″ × 2½″ pans.

Combine flour, xanthan gum, baking soda, baking powder, sugar, salt, and spice in mixing bowl. In another bowl, beat eggs. Add pumpkin and mayonnaise. Pour this into flour mixture. Stir all together well. Add pecans or dried fruit and pour into prepared pan(s). Bake the larger pan for 1 hour; or the smaller ones for about 45 to 50 minutes.

Nutrients per slice: Calories 100, Fat 4 g, Carbohydrate 14 g, Cholesterol 30 mg, Sodium 180 mg, Fiber 0, Protein 1 g

Small Breads

Quick and Easy Muffins 350°

These are a standby for me when I run out of bread. They take only one pan to mix and taste good both hot and cold. These come out best when mixed by hand with a mixing spoon.

¼ cup sugar
2 tablespoons shortening
2 eggs
1 cup GF Mix (page 38) or all rice flour
¼ teaspoon salt
¼ teaspoon xanthan gum
2 teaspoons baking powder
½ cup milk or nondairy liquid
¼ teaspoon vanilla

Preheat oven to 350°. Grease 8 muffin cups.

In the mixing bowl, cream together sugar and shortening. Then beat in the eggs.

Sift together the flour, salt, xanthan gum, and baking powder and add to the egg mixture alternately with the milk. Don't overbeat. Stir in the vanilla.

Pour into greased muffin cups. Bake for about 20 minutes. *Makes 8 muffins.*

Nutrients per muffin: Calories 150, Fat 5 g, Carbohydrate 23 g, Cholesterol 55 mg, Sodium 190 mg, Fiber 0, Protein 3 g

BLUEBERRY OR CRANBERRY MUFFINS: Add 1 to 1½ tablespoons blueberries or cranberries, fresh or frozen. (I keep these in a bag in the freezer and break apart what I need as I use them. It doesn't hurt the muffins to put them in still frozen.)

Muffin Mix (and More) 375°

Having mixes on hand can save a lot of kitchen time. This muffin mix will not only turn out muffins but can top a fruit cobbler or even make a quick cake. Keep it at home and take it along when you plan to stay with friends or in a place with a kitchen.

2½ cups rice flour
½ cup potato starch flour
½ cup tapioca flour
1 teaspoon baking soda
4 teaspoons baking powder
1 teaspoon salt
1 tablespoon Egg Replacer
1½ teaspoons xanthan gum
⅓ cup sugar
2 teaspoons dried lemon peel or powdered vanilla

Whisk together all the ingredients and store in an airtight container. *Makes enough for 4 batches of baking.*

To make muffins: Place 1 cup mix in a mixing bowl. In a small bowl, beat 2 eggs, 2 tablespoons vegetable oil or melted butter, and ⅓ cup liquid (buttermilk, milk, nondairy liquid, fruit juice, or carbonated drink). Pour into the flour mix and stir until smooth. Do not overbeat. Spoon into 6 greased muffin cups and bake in a preheated 375° oven for 12 to 15 minutes. *Makes 6 muffins.*

Nutrients per muffin: Calories 370, Fat 1 g, Carbohydrate 49 g, Cholesterol 0, Sodium 890 mg, Fiber 1 g, Protein 0

TO VARY TASTE: Add ¼ cup raisins, nuts, mashed bananas, chopped dates, or ⅓ cup grated fresh apple.

TO MAKE COBBLER: Mix as for muffins and drop the mix by spoonfuls atop 1 quart fresh berries or sliced peaches (that have been heated in 1½ cups water with sufficient sugar to sweeten) in an 8″ × 8″ pan. Bake in a preheated 350° oven for 20 to 25 minutes, or until the top is brown and springs back when lightly pressed.

TO MAKE AN 8-INCH SINGLE-LAYER ROUND CAKE: Mix as for muffins but add 1 more tablespoon sugar to 1 cup mix and spoon dough into a greased pan. Bake in a preheated 350° oven for 20 to 25 minutes. Serve with whipped cream and fruit, or frost to your taste.

Rice Bran Muffins 350°

This is a variation on Quick and Easy Muffins, but the bran changes the taste. I often add raisins to this batter.

¼ cup brown sugar
2 tablespoons shortening
2 eggs
⅔ cup brown rice flour
1 tablespoon tapioca flour
2 tablespoons potato starch flour
2 teaspoons baking powder
½ teaspoon xanthan gum
½ teaspoon salt
¾ cup milk or nondairy liquid
½ cup rice bran
¼ cup raisins (optional)

Preheat oven to 350°. Grease 8 muffin cups.

Cream together the sugar and shortening. Add the eggs, beating after each one.

Sift the flours together with the baking powder, xanthan gum, and salt. Add to the egg mixture alternately with the milk. Stir in rice bran last, then raisins if used.

Bake for 20 to 25 minutes. *Makes approximately 8 muffins.*

Nutrients per muffin: Calories 180, Fat 7 g, Carbohydrate 28 g, Cholesterol 55 mg, Sodium 270 mg, Fiber 1 g, Protein 4 g

Kasha (Buckwheat) Muffins 350°

This nutty-tasting variation of the bran muffin is an excellent change. Buckwheat contains no gluten, so celiacs should be able to eat this kasha form, thus getting more fiber into their diets.

⅓ cup brown sugar
2 tablespoons shortening
2 eggs
⅔ cup brown rice flour
1 tablespoon tapioca flour
2 tablespoons potato starch flour
2 teaspoons baking powder
¼ teaspoon xanthan gum
¾ cup milk
½ cup kasha (roasted buckwheat kernels)
1 teaspoon grated orange peel

Preheat oven to 350°. Grease 8 muffin cups.

Cream together the sugar and shortening. Add the eggs, beating after each one.

Sift the flours together with the baking powder and xanthan gum and add to the egg mixture alternately with the milk. Stir in buckwheat kernels and grated orange peel last.

Bake in prepared tins for 20 to 25 minutes. *Makes approximately 8 muffins.*

Nutrients per muffin: Calories 190, Fat 6 g, Carbohydrate 31 g, Cholesterol 55 mg, Sodium 125 mg, Fiber 1 g, Protein 5 g

Zucchini Muffins

400°

These spicy, tender muffins stay fresh-tasting and moist for several days because of the zucchini in the recipe. They are my favorite during the zucchini season.

⅓ cup sugar
2 eggs
3 tablespoons vegetable oil
1 cup GF Mix (page 38)
1 teaspoon baking powder
¾ teaspoon salt
½ teaspoon baking soda
¼ teaspoon cinnamon
¼ teaspoon nutmeg
1 cup grated zucchini
¼ cup raisins
¼ cup chopped walnuts

Preheat oven to 400°. Grease 10 to 12 muffin cups.

Beat together the sugar, eggs, and oil.

Combine the flour, baking powder, salt, baking soda, cinnamon, and nutmeg. Stir these into the sugar mixture. The batter will seem dry. Stir in the zucchini, raisins, and nuts.

Spoon batter into prepared cups to two-thirds full. Bake for 20 minutes. *Makes 10 to 12 muffins.*

Nutrients per muffin: Calories 130, Fat 5 g, Carbohydrate 19 g, Cholesterol 35 mg, Sodium 240 mg, Fiber 1 g, Protein 2 g

Spicy Carrot Muffins

425°

This is another muffin that stays moist. It's so good it's almost dessert.

1½ cups GF Mix (page 38)
½ cup rice bran
1 teaspoon cinnamon
¾ teaspoon baking soda
2 teaspoons baking powder
¼ teaspoon nutmeg
1 cup shredded carrots
⅔ cup orange juice
⅓ cup raisins
¼ cup vegetable oil
¼ cup brown sugar
2 eggs

Preheat oven to 425°. Grease 10 muffin cups or line with paper liners.

In a large bowl, combine flour, bran, cinnamon, baking soda, baking powder, and nutmeg. Mix well.

Combine carrots, orange juice, raisins, oil, brown sugar, and eggs and add to dry mixture, mixing until dry ingredients are moistened.

Spoon batter into prepared cups, filling about two-thirds. Let stand 5 minutes.

Bake 20 to 25 minutes. *Makes 10 muffins.*

Nutrients per muffin: Calories 290, Fat 18 g, Carbohydrate 31 g, Cholesterol 45 mg, Sodium 120 mg, Fiber 1 g, Protein 3 g

Buttermilk Biscuits

400°

Biscuits are more difficult to make with a rice flour base, since the cook does not usually have egg for leavening. But these (with the one egg added) have proved very good. They may be used as a bread substitute or as a base for creamed foods or berry shortcake.

1 tablespoon sugar
3 tablespoons shortening
1 egg
½ cup rice flour
⅓ cup potato starch flour
2 teaspoons baking powder
½ teaspoon baking soda
½ teaspoon salt
⅓ cup buttermilk

Preheat oven to 400°. Grease a baking sheet.

Mix the sugar, shortening, and egg. Sift the dry ingredients together and add them to the sugar mixture alternately with the buttermilk.

Pat out the mixture onto rice-floured wax paper and cut into round biscuit shapes. Or make drop biscuits by dropping the batter by tablespoonfuls onto a greased baking sheet.

Bake for 12 to 15 minutes. *Makes eight 2½-inch biscuits.*

Nutrients per biscuit: Calories 130, Fat 6 g, Carbohydrate 18 g, Cholesterol 25 mg, Sodium 320 mg, Fiber 0, Protein 2 g

Biscuit Mix

Keep this mix in a container in your refrigerator and have biscuits or a topping for your stew or chicken pie in minutes.

3 cups rice flour
2 cups potato starch flour
⅓ cup sugar
4 tablespoons baking powder
1 cup powdered buttermilk
1 tablespoon baking soda
1 tablespoon salt
1 cup plus 2 tablespoons shortening

In a large bowl, whisk together all the dry ingredients. Cut in the shortening until the mixture is crumbly. *Makes 6 batches of biscuits.*

TO MAKE BISCUITS: Add 1 beaten egg and ¼ cup water to 1¼ cups mix. Stir gently to moisten. Roll out onto a rice-floured board and cut into biscuit shapes. Bake in a preheated oven at 400° for 12 to 15 minutes. *Makes 8 to 10 biscuits.*

Nutrients per biscuit: Calories 130, Fat 6 g, Carbohydrate 18 g, Cholesterol 25 mg, Sodium 320 mg, Fiber 0, Protein 2 g

TO TOP COOKED STEWS OR CHICKEN PIES: Add 1 beaten egg and ⅓ cup water to 1¼ cups mix. Stir to moisten and drop by spoonfuls on the hot stew or pie. Bake at about 350° for 20–25 minutes, or until the biscuits are done.

Popovers

450°, 350°

Easy to make and impressive. This batter is very forgiving and always turns out.

1 cup water
½ cup shortening
⅓ cup potato starch flour
⅔ cup rice flour
½ teaspoon salt
4 eggs

Preheat oven to 450°. Grease 15 muffin cups.

Combine water and shortening in a large saucepan. Bring to a rapid boil. Remove from stove. Add flours and salt all at once. Stir until mixture forms a ball that leaves the sides of pan. Cool slightly. Add unbeaten eggs one at a time, beating well with electric mixer after each egg is added.

Drop by tablespoons into prepared cups to form a goose-egg-sized mound. Bake 20 minutes, then reduce heat and bake 20 minutes at 350°. *Makes about 15 popovers.*

Nutrients per roll: Calories 120, Fat 8 g, Carbohydrate 9 g, Cholesterol 55 mg, Sodium 90 mg, Fiber 0, Protein 2 g

Sugar-free White Corn Muffins

425°

I have included several cornbreads, but these are perhaps my favorites, for they come out moist and tasting a bit like hominy grits.

2 cups white cornmeal
1½ teaspoons salt
2 cups boiling water
2 eggs
2 tablespoons butter or margarine, melted
1 cup cold milk or nondairy liquid
4 teaspoons baking powder

Preheat oven to 425°. Grease 16 muffin cups.

In a large bowl, mix together the cornmeal and salt. Gradually stir in the boiling water. Beat with spoon until smooth.

Beat the eggs. Stir with the melted butter and milk into the flour mixture. Finally, stir in the baking powder.

Pour into prepared cups. Bake for 25 to 30 minutes. *Makes about 16 muffins.*

Nutrients per muffin: Calories 90, Fat 3 g, Carbohydrate 13 g, Cholesterol 35 mg, Sodium 240 mg, Fiber 2 g, Protein 3 g

Yellow Corn Muffins 400°

For an entirely different taste and texture from the preceding muffins, try these dry and fluffy ones.

1 cup yellow cornmeal
1 cup corn flour
¼ cup sugar
2 teaspoons baking powder
1 teaspoon baking soda
1 teaspoon salt
2 eggs, beaten
1 cup buttermilk
2 tablespoons shortening, melted

Preheat oven to 400°. Grease 12 muffin cups.

Sift the dry ingredients together into a mixing bowl. Stir in the beaten eggs, buttermilk, and melted shortening.

Spoon into prepared cups. Bake for about 25 minutes. *Makes about 12 muffins.*

Nutrients per muffin: Calories 130, Fat 4 g, Carbohydrate 22 g, Cholesterol 35 mg, Sodium 380 mg, Fiber 2 g, Protein 3 g

Orange Cornbread 400°

The use of fresh grated orange rind and corn flour instead of cornmeal makes this different in both texture and taste. This may be eaten hot from the oven as a bread, but try it other ways. It makes a great dressing for your Thanksgiving turkey (see page 195) and is perfect for stuffed pork chops or as a dressing beside a pork roast.

2 cups corn flour
2 tablespoons sugar
4 teaspoons baking powder
½ teaspoon salt
1 cup milk
3 eggs, beaten
⅓ cup vegetable oil
2 teaspoons grated orange peel

Preheat oven to 400°. Grease a 9″ × 9″ square baking pan.

In mixing bowl, combine corn flour, sugar, baking powder, and salt. Stir in milk, eggs, oil, and orange peel until smooth. Do not overbeat.

Pour into the prepared pan. Bake for 20 to 25 minutes. *Serves 6 to 8 as a cornbread or stuffs a 12- to 14-pound turkey.*

Nutrients per serving: Calories 250, Fat 13 g, Carbohydrate 28 g, Cholesterol 85 mg, Sodium 360 mg, Fiber 5 g, Protein 5 g

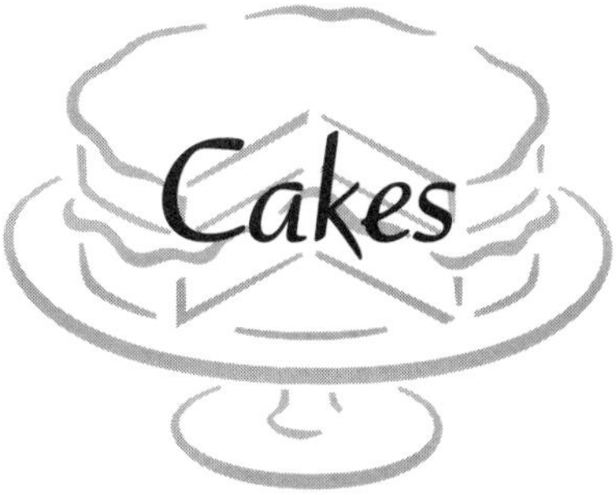

Cakes

Cheesecakes

Individual Cakes

Frostings

See Also

Some of today's homemakers are so used to cake mixes or picking up a cake in a bakery that starting from scratch may seem more effort than it is worth, but for anyone who cannot tolerate gluten, this is still the best way to have a cake and eat it, too. In the last decade several companies have created gluten-free cake mixes. Most of these are sold by phone or mail (see suppliers listed on pages 309–15), but a few are gradually finding a place on health food store or specialty grocery shelves. Within the next few years you may be able to pick up one of these while grocery shopping, but until then there are recipes in this section for almost any type of cake.

The recipes in this section have been selected because, in most instances, they are the easiest and the tastiest using our flours. They cover a wide range, from a simple white cake through the fruit and carrot cakes. For these cakes I use different combinations of flour.

For others I use one of my gluten-free flour mixes, which I keep on hand at all times.

Lemon Sheet Cake (Revised) 350°

When I first started baking, I almost despaired of making a successful basic cake. Now that I've discovered some of the secrets, I've found that simple cakes like this can come out fine-textured and moist with a delightful lemon flavor. This may be frosted, cut into shapes, and made into petit fours, or used as a shortcake with berries. This is a quick cake to mix. It can be doubled for a 9" by 13" oblong flat cake or two 9" round cake pans.

1 cup GF Mix (page 38) plus ¼ cup cornstarch
¾ teaspoon xanthan gum
1 teaspoon Egg Replacer
1 teaspoon unflavored gelatin
1 teaspoon baking soda
1 teaspoon baking powder
½ teaspoon salt
⅓ cup butter or margarine
¾ cup sugar
2 eggs
2 tablespoons lemon juice
1 tablespoon lemon zest
1 teaspoon vanilla
⅓ cup citrus-flavored soda drink

Preheat the oven to 350°. Grease an 8½" square cake pan and dust with rice flour.

In a medium bowl, whisk together the flour mix and cornstarch, xanthan gum, Egg Replacer, gelatin, baking soda, baking powder, and salt. Set aside.

In bowl of mixer, cream the butter and sugar. Beat in the eggs, one at a time, beating well after each addition. Add the lemon juice and zest.

Reduce mixer speed and add the dry ingredients alternately with the soda, beginning and ending with the dry ingredients. Beat until well incorporated but no more than 1 minute. Spoon into the prepared pan and bake at 350° for 25 to 30 minutes for the square pan, 35 to 40 minutes for the 9" × 13" oblong pan, and 20 to 25 for two round pans. Cake is done when a toothpick inserted in the center comes out clean and the cake pulls slightly from the pan edges. Cool before frosting. *Makes 8 to 9 servings.*

Nutrients per serving: Calories 250, Fat 9 g, Carbohydrate 37 g, Cholesterol 105 mg, Sodium 35 mg, Fiber 0, Protein 4 g

VARIATION: Add ¼ cup chopped nuts and ¼ cup raisins and serve as a coffee cake.

Pineapple or Peach Upside-down Cake

375°

This variation of the preceding cake is an old family favorite. The addition of the fruit topping saves making a frosting and keeps the cake more moist. This is especially tasty served hot from the oven.

1 recipe Lemon Sheet Cake (page 92)
⅓ cup (⅔ stick) butter or margarine
½ cup brown sugar
One 28-ounce can peach halves or pineapple slices, drained

Preheat oven to 375°. Instead of greasing the cake pan, use a combination of the butter and brown sugar melted together in the pan. Then arrange the pineapple or peach halves, cut sides down, in the sugar mixture. Prepare cake batter. Carefully spoon onto the peach halves.

Bake in 375° oven for 25 to 35 minutes. Serve in squares, fruit side up, topped with whipped cream. *Makes 6 to 8 servings.*

Nutrients per serving: Calories 190, Fat 5 g, Carbohydrate 28 g, Cholesterol 35 mg, Sodium 90 mg, Fiber 1 g, Protein 1 g

Classic Sponge Cake 300°

A fine-textured, springy cake with delicate flavor that is excellent eaten plain or with fruit. Or it can be glazed by drizzling on a thin mixture of butter, powdered sugar, and lemon juice. It keeps well.

½ cup rice flour
½ cup tapioca flour
¾ teaspoon baking powder
¼ teaspoon salt
7 eggs, separated
1 teaspoon grated lemon peel
¾ cup sugar
1 teaspoon cream of tartar

Preheat oven to 300°. Have handy a 9″ tube pan.

Sift together the flours, baking powder, and salt. Set aside.

Separate the eggs, placing the yolks in a 1½-quart bowl and the whites in a large mixing bowl. With mixer, whip the yolks on high speed for 3 to 5 minutes. Add the lemon peel and continue to whip until thick and pale yellow.

With clean beaters, whip the egg whites for 1 minute. Add 1 tablespoon sugar and the cream of tartar and continue whipping for 4 to 5 minutes, or until the whites are glossy and stiff. Remove mixer.

Pour the yolks onto the whites and gently fold together. Sprinkle about one-third of the remaining sugar over the surface and fold to incorporate. Add the rest in two more foldings. In the same way, in three additions, add the flour mixture, folding each time until just incorporated.

Pour the batter into the ungreased pan. Bake in 300° oven for about 50 to 60 minutes, or until the cake springs back when pressed with a finger.

To cool, turn the pan upside down and let stand for 2 hours before removing cake. (If your tube pan doesn't have raised "feet" around the rim, hang it by its tube over a soda bottle.)

Nutrients per serving: Calories 130, Fat 3 g, Carbohydrate 22 g, Cholesterol 125 mg, Sodium 105 mg, Fiber 0, Protein 4 g

Orange Chiffon Cake 325°, 350°

A fine, spongy cake that lasts—unless you let nonceliacs taste it. This is one of my favorite "company" cakes, for it doesn't taste grainy or dry out as fast as some nongluten baked products do. I drizzle this lightly with a frosting of powdered sugar, a bit of butter, and some orange juice, which I mix thin enough to pour easily. You might prefer to use a cream cheese frosting (page 114). The cake can also be served with whipped cream or an orange sauce, or used for strawberry shortcake.

If you wish, you may substitute 2 cups sifted GF Mix or Four Flour Bean Mix (pages 38–39) for the rice flour and potato starch flour.

1⅓ cups rice flour
⅔ cup potato starch flour
1½ cups sugar
1 tablespoon baking powder
1 teaspoon salt
½ cup vegetable oil
7 eggs, separated
¾ cup orange juice
2 teaspoons grated orange rind
½ teaspoon cream of tartar

Preheat oven to 325° for a large tube pan or 350° for 9″ × 13″ oblong cake pan.

Sift together into a mixing bowl the flours, sugar, baking powder, and salt. Make a well in the dry ingredients and add in order: oil, unbeaten egg yolks, orange juice, and rind. Beat together with a spoon until smooth.

In a large bowl, beat with electric mixer the egg whites and cream of tartar until they form very stiff peaks. Pour the egg yolk mixture gradually over the whipped whites, gently folding with a rubber scraper until just blended.

Pour batter into the tube pan or oblong pan. Bake tube pan at 325° for 55 minutes, then raise temperature to 350° for 10 to 15 minutes. Bake oblong pan at 350° for 45 to 50 minutes.

Nutrients per serving: Calories 170, Fat 6 g, Carbohydrate 25 g, Cholesterol 65 mg, Sodium 160 mg, Fiber 0, Protein 2 g

German Chocolate Cake 350°

Tender and moist, this is the perfect chocolate cake for all chocolate lovers. Serve it to guests; they'll never guess it isn't made with wheat flour.

2¼ cups Four Flour Bean Mix or GF Mix (pages 38–39)
1¼ teaspoons xanthan gum
1¼ teaspoons baking soda
1 teaspoon baking powder
1 teaspoon Egg Replacer
½ teaspoon salt.
4 squares (1 ounce each) semisweet chocolate
½ cup hot water
1 cup (2 sticks) margarine or butter
2 cups sugar
4 eggs
1 cup buttermilk
1 teaspoon vanilla

Preheat oven to 350°. Grease two 9″ cake pans or a 9″ × 13″ oblong pan and dust with rice flour.

In a medium bowl, whisk together the flour mix, xanthan gum, baking soda, baking powder, Egg Replacer, and salt. Set aside.

In a microwavable bowl, place the chocolate in the hot water and microwave on Defrost for 2 minutes. (Or place water and chocolate in a double boiler over boiling water. Stir until chocolate melts.) Set aside.

In mixing bowl, cream the margarine and sugar until fluffy. Add the eggs, one at a time, beating after each addition. Pour in chocolate and blend. Add the flour alternately with the buttermilk and vanilla in two additions. Beat on low speed until well blended. Spoon into prepared pan(s) and bake at 350° for 35 to 45 minutes. When cool, frost with Coconut-Pecan Frosting (page 116). *Makes 16 to 20 servings.*

Nutrients per serving: Calories 503, Fat 29 g, Carbohydrate 62 g, Cholesterol 145 mg, Sodium 480 mg, Fiber 2 g, Protein 6 g

Mock Black Forest Cake 350°

The flavor of this cake with its blend of chocolate, cherries, and liqueur is a winner with my friends. They don't even suspect it's gluten free. The rice, potato, and soy flours can be replaced by 1⅔ cups Four Flour Bean Mix (pages 38–39).

One 17-ounce can dark sweet cherries, pitted
2 tablespoons kirschwasser
6 tablespoons (¾ stick) butter or margarine
¾ cup sour cream or nondairy substitute
2 eggs, beaten
1 cup rice flour
½ cup potato starch flour
1 tablespoon soy flour
¾ cup sugar
2 teaspoons baking powder
½ teaspoon baking soda
½ teaspoon salt
2 squares semisweet baking chocolate

Preheat oven to 350°. Grease a 9″ × 5″ × 4″ loaf pan and dust with rice flour.

Drain cherries and slice into a small bowl. Cover with liqueur and let stand at least 10 minutes. Melt the butter and add it with the sour cream and eggs to the cherries. Blend well.

In a large bowl, combine flours, sugar, baking powder, baking soda, and salt. Add the cherry mixture and stir until moistened. Melt the chocolate and stir into cake batter.

Pour batter into prepared pan. Bake in 350° oven for 65 to 70 minutes. Cool cake in pan on wire rack for 15 minutes, then remove from pan and cool thoroughly.

Serve with whipped cream. Flavor increases if cake sits overnight.

Nutrients per serving: Calories 280, Fat 12 g, Carbohydrate 40 g, Cholesterol 55 mg, Sodium 280 mg, Fiber 1 g, Protein 3 g

Fruit Cocktail Torte

325°

A moist pudding cake that is quick, easy, and delicious. This may be served either hot or cold with whipped cream or whipped nondairy topping. My guests never guess it's gluten free.

1 cup GF Mix or Four Flour Bean Mix (pages 38–39)
1 cup sugar
1 teaspoon salt
1 teaspoon baking soda
2 eggs, beaten
One 17-ounce can fruit cocktail
1 teaspoon vanilla
½ cup brown sugar
½ cup chopped nuts

Preheat oven to 325°. Grease a 9″ × 9″ square cake pan and dust with rice flour.

In a mixing bowl, sift together the flour, sugar, salt, and baking soda.

Add the beaten eggs, fruit cocktail (juice included), and vanilla. Stir until well blended. Pour batter into the prepared pan and sprinkle with the brown sugar and nuts.

Bake at 325° for 1 hour. Serve warm or cold topped with whipped cream.

For variety, try coconut in place of the chopped nuts.

Nutrients per serving: Calories 180, Fat 3 g, Carbohydrate 38 g, Cholesterol 35 mg, Sodium 300 mg, Fiber 1 g, Protein 3 g

Katherine's Banana Cake with Meringue Frosting

350°

A super cake with a baked frosting. What could be easier? If you don't have buttermilk, use fresh milk clabbered with 2 teaspoons cider vinegar or lemon juice.

2 cups Four Flour Bean Mix or GF Mix (pages 38–39)
1 teaspoon xanthan gum
1½ teaspoons baking soda
2 teaspoons baking powder
¾ teaspoon salt
2 teaspoons Egg Replacer (optional)
1½ cups sugar
½ cup (1 stick) margarine or butter
2 eggs plus 1 egg white
1 teaspoon Vanilla, Butter, and Nut flavoring or vanilla flavoring
1 cup mashed bananas
1 tablespoon lemon juice
½ cup buttermilk
½ cup chopped walnuts or pecans (optional)

Preheat oven to 350°. Grease a 9″ × 13″ oblong cake pan and dust with rice flour.

In a medium bowl, combine the flour mix, xanthan gum, baking soda, baking powder, salt, and Egg Replacer (if used). Set aside.

In the bowl of your mixer, cream the sugar and margarine. Beat in the eggs and egg white until well blended and light. Add the flavoring and mix well. Blend in the bananas (with the lemon juice stirred in) and the buttermilk alternately in 2 additions. Beat for about 1 minute. Remove bowl from mixing stand and stir in the nuts (if using), reserving 2 tablespoons for the topping. Spoon batter into prepared pan and cover with the following meringue.

Meringue: Beat 1 egg white until it forms stiff peaks. Slowly add ½ cup brown sugar. Spread in a thin layer across the top of the unbaked batter. Sprinkle with about 2 tablespoons chopped nuts. Bake at 350° for approximately 45 minutes.

Nutrients per serving: Calories 160, Fat 6 g, Carbohydrate 25 g, Cholesterol 30 mg, Sodium 230 mg, Fiber 1 g, Protein 2 g

Lemon Pound Cake

325°

This simple but versatile cake can have just a hint of lemon without the glaze. Use the glaze for a strong lemon flavor. Serve this plain or top it with fresh fruit. The texture will be like a wheat cake with the Four Flour Mix but a bit more grainy with the rice-based GF Mix.

2¼ cups Four Flour Bean Mix or GF Mix (pages 38–39)
1⅛ teaspoons xanthan gum
1 teaspoon Egg Replacer (optional)
1 teaspoon salt
1¼ cups sugar
1 tablespoon grated lemon peel
⅔ cup butter or margarine
½ cup milk
1 tablespoon lemon juice
3 eggs

GLAZE
½ cup sugar
¼ cup lemon juice

Preheat oven to 325°. Grease a 9″ × 5″ × 3″ loaf pan and dust with rice flour.

In the bowl of your mixer, place flour mix, xanthan gum, Egg Replacer (if used), salt, sugar, and lemon peel. Make a well in the center and add the butter and milk. Stir to combine. Scrape bowl, turn to low speed, and beat 1 minute.

Add lemon juice and eggs. Beat on low for about 30 seconds. Scrape bowl down again. Turn to medium speed and beat 1 minute or until fluffy. Spoon batter into prepared pan and bake for 1 hour and 10 minutes. Cool in pan a few minutes before turning out. Glaze while still hot.

To glaze: In a saucepan, heat sugar and lemon juice to boiling. Brush on cake while still warm. The cake should absorb all the glaze. *Makes 12 to 16 servings.*

Nutrients per serving: Calories 250, Fat 9 g, Carbohydrate 41 g, Cholesterol 60 mg, Sodium 230 mg, Fiber 0, Protein 2 g

Zucchini Cake

350°

This easy-to-stir-up cake stays moist for days. The bean flour mix plus the zucchini and spice make the flavor so delicious you can offer this to any guest. This recipe may be halved for an 8" square cake pan.

2½ cups Four Flour Bean Mix or GF Mix (pages 38–39)
1 rounded teaspoon xanthan gum
2 teaspoons Egg Replacer (optional)
2 cups sugar
2 teaspoons cinnamon
1 teaspoon salt
2 teaspoons baking powder
1 teaspoon baking soda
4 eggs
1 cup vegetable oil
2 cups grated zucchini
½ cup chopped walnuts

Preheat oven to 350°. Grease a 9" × 13" oblong baking pan.

In a mixing bowl, combine the flour mix, xanthan gum, Egg Replacer (if used), sugar, cinnamon, salt, baking powder, and baking soda.

In a medium bowl, beat the eggs until fluffy and lemon colored. Add the oil and beat another 2 minutes. Pour this into the dry ingredients and mix well. Add the zucchini and stir until thoroughly combined. Fold in the walnuts.

Spoon into the prepared pan and bake at 350° for 35 to 40 minutes, or until a tester inserted near the center comes out clean. Cool before frosting with your favorite cream cheese or vanilla icing. *Makes 12 to 15 servings.*

Nutrients per serving: Calories 350, Fat 18 g, Carbohydrate 46 g, Cholesterol 55 mg, Sodium 300 mg, Fiber 1 g, Protein 4 g

Carrot Cake Supreme 350°

The use of fruit or carrots in a cake almost always ensures success for the gluten-free flours, especially if you use soy flour along with the rice flours. But this cake is even tastier than other recipes I tried. The secret ingredient is the mayonnaise. You may replace the rice, soy, and potato starch flours with 2½ cups Four Flour Bean Mix (pages 38–39).

1½ cups rice flour
½ cup soy flour
½ cup potato starch flour
1 teaspoon xanthan gum
2 teaspoons baking soda
2 teaspoons cinnamon
½ teaspoon powdered ginger
½ teaspoon salt
4 large eggs
2 cups sugar
1 cup mayonnaise
One 16-ounce can crushed pineapple
3 cups grated carrots
1 cup chopped walnuts

In a bowl, stir together the flours, xanthan gum, baking soda, cinnamon, ginger, and salt. Set aside.

In large bowl of the mixer, beat together at medium speed the eggs, sugar, mayonnaise, and pineapple, not drained. Gradually beat in flour mixture until well mixed. With a spoon, stir in carrots and walnuts.

Pour batter into a greased and rice-floured 9″ × 13″ pan. Bake in preheated 350° oven for 45 to 50 minutes, or until cake tester inserted in the center comes out clean. Cool in pan.

Serve with whipped cream or frost with cream cheese frosting. *Makes 16 servings.*

Nutrients per serving: Calories 240, Fat 11 g, Carbohydrate 35 g, Cholesterol 40 mg, Sodium 220 mg, Fiber 1 g, Protein 3 g

Apple Raisin Cake

350°

A moist, fruity cake that keeps well. The chopped apples and the soy flour add to its moistness. Like the carrot cake, this uses mayonnaise instead of oil or shortening. You may replace the rice, soy, and potato starch flours with 2½ cups Four Flour Bean Mix (pages 38–39)

2 cups rice flour
½ cup soy flour
2 tablespoons potato starch flour
1¼ teaspoons xanthan gum
2 cups sugar
1 cup mayonnaise
⅓ cup milk or nondairy substitute
3 eggs
2 rounded teaspoons baking soda
1½ teaspoons cinnamon
½ teaspoon nutmeg
¼ teaspoon ground cloves
½ teaspoon salt
3 cups chopped peeled apples
1 cup raisins
½ cup chopped walnuts

Preheat oven to 350°. Grease a 9″ × 13″ oblong cake pan and dust with rice flour.

Place in a large mixing bowl the flours, xanthan gum, sugar, mayonnaise, milk, eggs, baking soda, spices, and salt. Beat with a mixer at low speed for 2 minutes, or 300 strokes by hand. Batter will be very thick.

Stir in apples, raisins, and nuts. Spoon batter into prepared pan. Bake at 350° for 45 minutes, or until a tester inserted in the center comes out clean. Cool in pan.

Serve with whipped cream or frost with cream cheese frosting. *Makes 16 servings.*

Nutrients per serving: Calories 240, Fat 10 g, Carbohydrate 39 g, Cholesterol 30 mg, Sodium 210 mg, Fiber 1 g, Protein 3 g

Raisin Rum Cake 350°

This is a real party cake with a rich rum flavor that will please a crowd. Remember to put the raisins to soak in the rum overnight. You may replace the rice and tapioca flours with 2½ cups Four Flour Bean Mix.

1 cup light raisins
⅓ cup dark rum
2 cups rice flour
½ cup tapioca flour
4 teaspoons baking powder
1½ teaspoons baking soda
½ teaspoon salt
¼ teaspoon nutmeg
2 teaspoons xanthan gum
1 cup mayonnaise
1 cup sugar
3 eggs
1 cup buttermilk
1 tablespoon grated lemon peel
1 tablespoon grated orange peel

RUM SAUCE
½ cup sugar
¼ cup water
2 tablespoons orange juice
2 tablespoons lemon juice
2 tablespoons dark rum
2 tablespoons powdered sugar (optional)

Soak the raisins in the rum overnight in a covered bowl until they are plump with rum and there is no moisture left in the bowl.

Preheat oven to 350°. Grease a bundt pan with 10–12-cup capacity and dust with rice flour.

Sift together the flours, baking powder, baking soda, salt, nutmeg, and xanthan gum. Set aside. In mixer bowl, place mayonnaise, sugar, and eggs. Beat together on medium speed for a few seconds, until the eggs are well beaten.

On low speed, add the dry ingredients in 3 additions, alternating with the buttermilk. Then, by hand, stir in the grated lemon and orange peels and rum-soaked raisins.

Pour batter into prepared pan. Bake for approximately 50 minutes, or until the cake tests done. Let the cake stand in the pan for 10 minutes before turning it out onto a cake plate. Add the rum sauce. *Makes 20 servings.*

Rum Sauce

In a small saucepan, boil together the sugar and water for 2 minutes. Remove from heat and stir in the orange juice, lemon juice, and rum. Using a pastry brush, brush the warm rum sauce over the warm cake. Let cool. Sprinkle the top with powdered sugar if desired.

Nutrients per serving: Calories 420, Fat 18 g, Carbohydrate 60 g, Cholesterol 60 mg, Sodium 510 mg, Fiber 2 g, Protein 5 g

Angel Food Cake

375°

An angel-light cake with a delicate mix of flours. I almost gave up on this one until I hit upon this successful formula.

7 egg whites (¾ cup)
½ cup powdered sugar
¼ cup potato starch flour
¼ cup cornstarch
⅓ cup granulated sugar
¾ teaspoon cream of tartar
¼ teaspoon salt
1 teaspoon dried lemon peel

Preheat the oven to 375°.

Set the egg whites aside to bring to room temperature.

Sift together into a small bowl the powdered sugar, flour, and cornstarch. The sifting is essential in this recipe. Measure the granulated sugar to have handy.

In a large glass or metal (not plastic) mixing bowl, place egg whites, cream of tartar, salt, and lemon peel. With mixer at high, beat until the mixture is well blended. Continue to beat while adding the granulated sugar slowly. Beat just until sugar is dissolved and whites form stiff peaks.

With a rubber spatula, gently fold in the flour and powdered sugar mixture about one-fourth at a time, folding just enough so the flour disappears.

Pour batter into ungreased 9″ tube pan and cut through with spatula to break any air bubbles. Bake at 375° for 35 minutes, or until top springs back when lightly touched. Remove from oven and cool cake in the inverted pan. Remove cake only when completely cool. *Makes 8 servings.*

This recipe can be doubled for a large 10″ tube pan.

Nutrients per serving: Calories 70, Fat 0, Carbohydrate 15 g, Cholesterol 0, Sodium 80 mg, Fiber 0, Protein 2 g

Cheesecakes

These are so easy to make that no cook should be afraid to try. I give three different cheesecake recipes; all can use the following crust.

CRUST

2 cups GF cereal or GF dried bread or cookie crumbs
3 tablespoons melted butter or margarine
2 tablespoons sugar
¼ teaspoon cinnamon
¼ teaspoon nutmeg

Crush the cereal or crumbs, add remaining ingredients, and mix together in a bowl or shake together in a plastic bag. Pat out into a 10″ springform pan or large pie plate, reserving a tablespoon to top the cheesecake before baking, if desired.

Simply Scrumptious Cheesecake

375°

A rich, never-fail cheesecake that can be eaten alone or with a topping of simple crushed fruit, either fresh or canned.

Three 8-ounce packages cream cheese
4 eggs
1 cup sugar
1 teaspoon vanilla

Preheat oven to 375°. Prepare the crust in a 10″ springform pan.

Soften cream cheese and combine with eggs, sugar, and vanilla. Beat with electric mixer until well blended. Pour into prepared crust and top with remaining crumb mixture. Bake for 35 to 40 minutes, or until set.

When cool, refrigerate several hours before serving with or without toppings. This is a large cake and very rich. *Serves 12.*

For a lighter version of this cake, use two 8-ounce packages cream cheese and 1 cup cottage cheese.

Nutrients per serving (includes cereal crust): Calories 300, Fat 22 g, Carbohydrate 20 g, Cholesterol 135 mg, Sodium 210 mg, Fiber 0, Protein 6 g

Orange Cheesecake

375°

A nice blend of flavors for both orange and cheesecake lovers. This is a smaller recipe than the preceding one so you can cut the crust mixture in half and pat into a small (9″) pie plate.

Two 3-ounce packages cream cheese
1 egg
⅓ cup sugar
⅓ cup sour cream or nondairy substitute
1 teaspoon grated orange peel
3 tablespoons orange juice
¼ teaspoon vanilla
¼ cup orange marmalade for topping

Preheat oven to 375°. Prepare crust in a 9″ pie plate.

Soften the cream cheese. Place in mixing bowl and blend with egg, sugar, and sour cream until the mixture is smooth. Add orange peel, orange juice, and vanilla.

Pour the mixture into prepared crust and bake in preheated 375° oven for about 30 to 35 minutes, or until set. Remove from oven and cool slightly while heating the marmalade in a saucepan or in microwave for ½ to 1 minute. Spoon this over top of cheesecake and refrigerate at least 3 hours. *Makes 6 servings.*

Nutrients per serving (includes cereal crust): Calories 240, Fat 14 g, Carbohydrate 26 g, Cholesterol 75 mg, Sodium 140 mg, Fiber 1 g, Protein 3 g

Linda's Lighter Cheesecake

A very light cheesecake with delicate fruit flavors. This is a large recipe so prepare two 8″ square pans or one 9″ × 13″ oblong pan with crust mixture suggested previously, again, reserving some for topping. Since this is a no-bake cheesecake, you can put the crust in a preheated oven at 375° for about 5 to 7 minutes to brown slightly, though it is not necessary.

One 6-ounce package lemon gelatin (see Note)
1 cup hot water
One 9-ounce can crushed pineapple (see Note)
16 ounces large-curd cottage cheese (low-fat is fine)
1 cup dry milk powder
½ cup ice water
3 tablespoons lemon juice
½ cup sugar
1½ to 2 tablespoons grated lemon rind

Keep ingredients cold at all times.

Dissolve gelatin in hot water and chill until slightly thickened.

Meanwhile, drain pineapple and reserve juice. Beat cottage cheese with electric mixer at low speed until very creamy. When gelatin has thickened, beat cottage cheese into gelatin and place in refrigerator.

Mix milk powder, ice water, and lemon juice. Beat until fluffy and stiff. Combine with slightly thickened gelatin and cheese mixture and beat at high speed. Add pineapple juice and sugar slowly, beating thoroughly. Fold in pineapple and lemon rind. Pour over crumb crust and top with remaining crumbs. Chill in refrigerator 2 to 4 hours. *Makes 15 servings.*

NOTE: Orange or peach gelatin may be used, and other fresh fruit may be substituted for the pineapple, but do not substitute fresh pineapple for canned, or the gelatin will not set.

Nutrients per serving (includes cereal crust): Calories 90, Fat 2.5 g, Carbohydrate 9 g, Cholesterol 10 mg, Sodium 270 mg, Fiber 0, Protein 7 g

Easy Mini Cheesecakes 325°

Use a thin GF cookie for the base and pour your cheesecake batter into a muffin tin for individual cheesecakes. Use either a purchased cookie or a home-baked gingersnap or sugar cookie or one made from the Refrigerator Roll recipe (page 137). These cheesecakes may be topped with the nuts as suggested in the recipe or made plain and decorated with a berry, a piece of fruit, or a few chocolate curls. If you offer these on a tray, you may want to make several different toppings for variety.

NOTE: Always check to be sure that your light cheese and sour cream are gluten free.

12 GF cookies
½ cup sugar
Two 8-ounce packages fat-reduced cream cheese, softened
2 eggs
2 teaspoons vanilla flavoring, separated
One 8-ounce carton light sour cream
2 tablespoons sugar
2 tablespoons chopped nuts for topping

Preheat oven to 325°. Line 12 muffin cups with foil liners. Place a cookie in each liner.

In the bowl of your mixer, combine the ½ cup sugar, cream cheese, eggs, and 1 teaspoon vanilla. Beat at medium speed until smooth. Spoon over each cookie, filling each cup about three-fourths full. Bake for 30 minutes.

Meanwhile, in a small bowl, stir together the sour cream, 2 tablespoons sugar, and the remaining teaspoon vanilla. Divide evenly by spooning about 1 tablespoon onto each hot mini cheesecake. Sprinkle chopped nuts evenly on top, return to oven, and continue baking for 8 to 10 minutes, or until set. Allow to cool thoroughly before removing from muffin tins. When cool, refrigerate to chill for 1 to 2 hours. If not serving immediately, keep refrigerated. Can be made a day ahead. *Makes 12 servings.*

Nutrients per serving: Calories 310, Fat 17 g, Carbohydrate 32 g, Cholesterol 75 mg, Sodium 370 mg, Fiber 0, Protein 6 g

Individual Cakes

Cream Puffs

450°, 350°

Don't be put off by the elegance of this dessert. It is one of the easiest to make with our flours. Try it and impress your guests.

1 cup water
½ cup shortening
⅓ cup potato starch flour
⅔ cup rice flour
½ teaspoon salt
1 tablespoon sugar
4 eggs

Preheat oven to 450°. Grease a cookie sheet.

Combine water and shortening in a large saucepan. Bring to a rapid boil. Mix flours, salt, and sugar and add to water and shortening. Stir until mixture forms a ball that leaves the sides of the pan. Remove from heat and cool slightly.

Add the unbeaten eggs, one at a time, beating well with electric mixer after each egg is added.

Drop by tablespoonfuls onto prepared cookie sheet. The puffs should be approximately 2 inches round and about 1½ inches high. Leave space for them to expand. Bake in 450° oven for 20 minutes, then reduce heat to 350° and bake for 20 minutes more. Remove from oven and prick with a knife to let steam escape.

Serve cold, filled with sweetened whipped cream. *Makes 8 to 10 puffs.*

Nutrients per puff: Calories 180, Fat 12 g, Carbohydrate 15 g, Cholesterol 85 mg, Sodium 135 mg, Fiber 0, Protein 4 g

Chocolate Eclairs

Another chou pastry dessert sure to please all guests. These can be made ahead and filled just before serving. Bake cream puff dough in elongated (finger) shapes by molding with damp rubber spatula or pressing out of a pastry bag.

1 recipe Cream Puffs, page 111

FILLING

1 cup cream or nondairy substitute
3 egg yolks
¼ cup sugar
3 tablespoons sweet rice flour
1 tablespoon butter or margarine
1 tablespoon rum

GLAZE

2 ounces semisweet chocolate
1 tablespoon coffee
1½ tablespoons butter or margarine

Heat the cream but do not boil. Set aside.

In a saucepan, whip egg yolks and gradually beat in sugar. Continue beating until mixture is thick and lemon colored. Slowly add flour, then heated cream.

Put saucepan over moderate heat and cook, stirring slowly, until the custard comes to a boil. If it starts to lump, beat vigorously. Cook about 3 minutes.

Remove from heat. Stir in butter and rum. Chill covered with plastic wrap to keep a skin from forming on the surface. Stir before filling the eclairs. (Do this 4 hours or less before serving so the eclairs will not become soggy.)

For the glaze, melt the chocolate and beat in the coffee and butter. Spread lightly on the eclairs. *Makes 8 to 10 eclairs.*

Nutrients per eclair: Calories 320, Fat 21 g, Carbohydrate 26 g, Cholesterol 165 mg, Sodium 180 mg, Fiber 1 g, Protein 6 g

Pecan Brownie Cupcakes

350°

These rich, fudgy brownies are baked as cupcakes, which keeps them moist. The single serving size is great for freezing for lunches or serving in single portions to the dieter. For the true chocoholic, ice with the chocolate frosting on page 114.

3 ounces unsweetened baking chocolate
¾ cup (1½ sticks) butter or margarine
1 cup brown sugar
½ cup granulated sugar
3 large eggs
1 teaspoon vanilla
¾ cup GF Mix (page 38)
1 cup chopped pecans
16 to 18 pecan halves for garnish (optional)

Preheat oven to 350°. Line 16 to 18 muffin cups with paper liners.

In a 2- or 3-quart saucepan, combine chocolate and butter. Place over low heat and stir occasionally until melted. Remove from heat. Stir in brown and granulated sugars. Beat in eggs, one at a time. Add vanilla. Beat in flour. Stir in chopped nuts.

Spoon batter into prepared muffin cups, filling about two-thirds full. If desired, place a pecan half on top of each. Bake at 350° for 22 to 25 minutes. Tops should look crackly, but interiors should still be slightly moist. Let cool in pan for 15 minutes, then remove and let cool on rack. *Makes 16 to 18 cupcakes.*

Nutrients per serving: Calories 230, Fat 16 g, Carbohydrate 21 g, Cholesterol 55 mg, Sodium 90 mg, Fiber 1 g, Protein 2 g

Cream Cheese Frosting ✓

There are several prepared cream cheese frostings on the market that are gluten free. But this is simple to make if you haven't a packaged one on hand.

One 8-ounce package cream cheese, softened
½ cup (1 stick) butter or margarine, softened
1 teaspoon vanilla
1 pound confectioner's sugar

Combine cream cheese, butter, and vanilla in a mixing bowl. Blend at low speed with electric mixer. Gradually add confectioner's sugar, beating until fluffy. You may add a few drops of cream, if necessary, to make spreading easier.

This makes a large recipe, enough for the tops of two 9″ × 13″ oblong cakes, but the frosting keeps in the refrigerator for days. Or better yet, freeze the balance for the next cake.

Nutrients per serving: Calories 140, Fat 7 g, Carbohydrate 19 g,
Cholesterol 20 mg, Sodium 70 mg, Fiber 0, Protein 0

Easy Chocolate Icing

Again, you may buy gluten-free chocolate frosting on the market, but this is an easy one. It keeps well in the refrigerator for several days and freezes well. Warm to room temperature to spread on cake or cupcakes.

4 squares semisweet baking chocolate
½ cup (1 stick) butter or margarine
1 pound confectioner's sugar
1 teaspoon vanilla
½ cup milk (approximately)

Melt chocolate in a saucepan over very low heat, stirring constantly. (Or melt in microwave in a glass bowl.)

Stir butter to soften. Beat in half the sugar. Blend in the chocolate and vanilla. Add the remaining sugar alternately with the milk, beating until smooth and of the right consistency to spread. *Makes 2½ cups icing.*

Nutrients per serving: Calories 130, Fat 6 g, Carbohydrate 21 g, Cholesterol 10 mg, Sodium 40 mg, Fiber 1 g, Protein 1 g

Penuche Frosting

This butterscotch-tasting frosting is especially good on spice or chocolate cakes. It's a bit more trouble than the preceding two but well worth it.

2 cups brown sugar
½ cup milk or nondairy liquid
½ cup (1 stick) margarine

Place ingredients in a saucepan and stir over low heat until margarine is melted. Bring rapidly to a full boil, stirring constantly. Boil to 220° on a candy thermometer, or exactly 1 minute. Remove from heat.

Beat until lukewarm and of the right consistency to spread. If frosting gets too hard, it can be thinned with a little cream. *Makes approximately 1½ cups icing or enough for 1 cake.*

Nutrients per serving: Calories 210, Fat 8 g, Carbohydrate 36 g, Cholesterol 20 mg, Sodium 95 mg, Fiber 0, Protein 0

Coconut-Pecan Frosting

This frosting, usually used on German chocolate cakes, dresses up any other chocolate cake. This may be found on grocery shelves but often contains gluten, so it's safer to make your own. Cut the recipe by one-third if frosting only the top of a 9" × 13" oblong cake.

1 cup evaporated milk
1 cup sugar
3 egg yolks, lightly beaten
½ cup (1 stick) butter or margarine
1 teaspoon vanilla
1⅓ cups flaked coconut
1 cup chopped pecans

In a medium saucepan, combine milk, sugar, egg yolks, butter, and vanilla. Stir while cooking over medium heat until thickened. Remove from heat and stir in coconut and pecans. Beat until frosting is cool and reaches desired spreading consistency. *Makes approximately 3 cups, which fills and frosts a two-layer cake.*

Nutrients per serving (2 tablespoons): Calories 110, Fat 8 g, Carbohydrate 10 g, Cholesterol 35 mg, Sodium 70 mg, Fiber 0, Protein 1 g

Cookies

Drop Cookies

Bar Cookies

Shaped Cookies

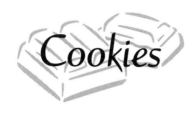

Cookies are probably the easiest baked item to make from gluten-free flours, and the results are almost always satisfying.

In the following pages you'll find a wide range of cookies that have turned out successfully in my kitchen. They range from the Chewy Fruit Bars that remind you of Christmas fruitcake to Butterscotch Chip Dreams you will have to hide from the rest of the family to have any for the celiac. There's even one nonbake recipe easy enough for children to make.

Some of these travel better than others. Those I carry on trips to have a sweet when others have a gluten-filled dessert.

Each recipe calls for a different combination of flours. Many use a combination of rice and soy, some call for the GF Mix suggested earlier, and others the Four Flour Bean Mix.

Butterscotch Bites

375°

An easy-to-make drop cookie that tastes great. These keep well in the cookie jar at home but don't travel as well as some of the other cookies, since they are moist and chewy and tend to stick together when bumped around. The rice and soy flours may be replaced by 1 cup Four Flour Bean Mix.

½ cup (1 stick) butter or margarine
1 cup dark brown sugar
1 egg
½ cup rice flour
½ cup soy flour
½ cup chopped pecans

Preheat oven to 375°.

Beat butter and sugar together until creamy. Beat in egg, then flours. Stir in nuts.

Drop by teaspoonfuls onto ungreased cookie sheets. Bake for 10 to 12 minutes. Remove immediately from baking sheet and let cool on wax paper. Store loosely covered. *Makes approximately 3 dozen cookies.*

Nutrients per cookie: Calories 60, Fat 4 g, Carbohydrate 7 g, Cholesterol 15 mg, Sodium 40 mg, Fiber 0, Protein 1 g

Butterscotch Chip Dreams

350°

A rich, moist cookie that will surprise your gluten-eating friends. This cookie keeps well for the lunch box. I like them made with butterscotch chips, but you may substitute chocolate chips or peanut butter chips.

1 cup (2 sticks) butter or margarine
1 cup brown sugar
2 eggs
1 teaspoon vanilla
2 cups soy flour
¼ cup rice flour
1 teaspoon baking soda
½ teaspoon salt
One 12-ounce package butterscotch chips

Preheat oven to 350°.

In a large bowl, beat with an electric mixer the butter, brown sugar, eggs, and vanilla. Combine the flours, baking soda, and salt and add to the creamed mixture. Stir in the chips.

Drop by teaspoonfuls onto ungreased cookie sheets. Bake for about 10 minutes. *Makes approximately 3 dozen cookies.*

Nutrients per cookie: Calories 130, Fat 9 g, Carbohydrate 10 g, Cholesterol 40 mg, Sodium 180 mg, Fiber 1 g, Protein 4 g

Peanut Butter Drops

350°

No, I didn't forget the flour in this one. The recipe doesn't call for any. Since this is a cookie that keeps and travels well, it's great for that quick energy snack on trips.

2 eggs
1 cup chunky peanut butter
1 cup sugar

Preheat oven to 350°

Beat the eggs. Stir in the peanut butter and sugar.

Drop by small spoonfuls on ungreased cookie sheets. Bake for 10 to 12 minutes. *Makes approximately 2½ dozen 2-inch cookies.*

Nutrients per cookie: Calories 80, Fat 5 g, Carbohydrate 9 g, Cholesterol 15 mg, Sodium 45 mg, Fiber 1 g, Protein 3 g

Forgotten Dreams 350°–0°

A meringue cookie that tastes more like candy than cookie. Easy to make. Can be made late at night and left in the oven overnight.

2 egg whites
⅛ teaspoon salt
½ teaspoon cream of tartar
½ cup sugar
½ teaspoon vanilla
6 ounces butterscotch or peanut butter chips

Preheat oven to 350°. Grease 2 cookie sheets.

With electric mixer, beat egg whites until foamy. Add salt and cream of tartar. Beat until whites form stiff peaks.

Add sugar gradually while beating. Beat in vanilla. Fold in the chips. Drop by teaspoonfuls on prepared sheets. Put in oven. Turn oven off and forget for 2 hours or more. *Makes about 60 small cookies.*

Nutrients per cookie: Calories 20, Fat 1 g, Carbohydrate 3 g, Cholesterol 5 mg, Sodium 65 mg, Fiber 0, Protein 1 g

Coconut Macaroons 350°

Although we can sometimes find GF macaroons on the cookie shelf in the supermarket, these are far tastier than any store-bought cookies and contain no flour.

½ teaspoon salt
4 egg whites
1¼ cups fine granulated sugar
1 teaspoon vanilla
2 cups sweetened shredded coconut

Preheat oven to 350°. Fit brown paper on 2 cookie sheets.

Add salt to egg whites and beat with electric mixer until stiff but not dry. Add sugar slowly, beating until granules are dissolved. Gently stir in vanilla and coconut. Drop by teaspoonfuls onto prepared cookie sheets.

Bake at 350° for about 20 minutes. Slip paper onto wet table or board and let stand for 1 minute. Loosen cookies and remove to wire racks. *Makes approximately 2½ dozen macaroons.*

Nutrients per cookie: Calories 60, Fat 2 g, Carbohydrate 11 g, Cholesterol 0, Sodium 60 mg, Fiber 0, Protein 1 g

Pecan Bites

300°

Another cookie more like candy than cookie. Like the preceding recipe, it contains no flour.

3 egg whites
3 cups light brown sugar
3 cups chopped pecans
¼ teaspoon salt
1 teaspoon vanilla

Preheat oven to 300°. Grease 2 cookie sheets.

Beat egg whites to soft peaks. Stir in the rest of the ingredients. Drop by scant tablespoonfuls onto prepared cookie sheets. Bake at 300° for about 20 minutes. *Makes approximately 6 dozen cookies.*

Nutrients per cookie: Calories 50, Fat 3 g, Carbohydrate 7 g, Cholesterol 0, Sodium 45 mg, Fiber 0, Protein 1 g

Carrot Raisin Drop Cookies

350°

These tender cookies are studded with raisins and nuts. The carrots give moistness; the cereal adds fiber. The cookies keep well—if you hide them away. The flour mix and soy flour may be replaced with 1½ cups Four Flour Bean Mix (pages 38–39).

1 cup GF Mix (page 38)
½ cup soy flour
1 rounded teaspoon baking soda
2 teaspoons pumpkin pie spice
1½ cups crushed GF cereal
½ cup (1 stick) butter or margarine
3 large eggs
1 cup corn syrup
2 cups grated carrots
1 cup raisins
½ cup chopped walnuts

Preheat oven to 350°. Grease 2 cookie sheets.

In a bowl, mix together flours, baking soda, spice, and GF cereal.

In another bowl, beat butter, eggs, and corn syrup with an electric mixer until blended. Mix in the carrots. Add the flour mixture. Stir until mixed, then beat until blended. Stir in raisins and nuts.

Spoon dough in tablespoon-sized mounds 2 inches apart on prepared cookie sheets. Bake until cookies feel firm when touched, 12 to 14 minutes. Remove from pans and cool. *Makes about 4 dozen cookies.*

Nutrients per cookie: Calories 80, Fat 3 g, Carbohydrate 13 g, Cholesterol 20 mg, Sodium 65 mg, Fiber 0, Protein 1 g

Chewy Oatmeal Cookies

375°

The oatmeal texture comes from soy flakes (which may be obtained from several of the mail-order suppliers). The chew comes from the raisins and zucchini. These cookies keep and travel well, and since they are not a sweet cookie, they are great for that after-school snack.

2¼ cups Four Flour Bean Mix (pages 38–39)
1 teaspoon xanthan gum
1 rounded teaspoon baking soda
1½ teaspoons cinnamon
¼ teaspoon ground cloves
¼ teaspoon salt
½ cup (1 stick) margarine or butter
¾ cup honey
1 egg
1 cup grated zucchini
1 cup soy flakes
1 cup raisins
1 cup chopped walnuts or pecans

Preheat oven to 375°. Grease a cookie sheet.

In a medium bowl, whisk together the flour, xanthan gum, baking soda, cinnamon, cloves, and salt. Set aside.

In the bowl of your mixer, cream the margarine with the honey. Add the egg and beat well. Add the dry ingredients alternately with the zucchini. Stir in the soy flakes, raisins, and nuts. Drop by rounded teaspoonfuls onto prepared cookie sheet. Bake at 375° for 10 to 12 minutes. *Makes 4½ dozen cookies.*

Nutrients per cookie: Calories 47, Fat 1½ g, Carbohydrate 8 g, Cholesterol 5 mg, Sodium 45 mg, Fiber 2 g, Protein 1 g

Cornflake Cookies 325°

Crisp, crunchy, and full of flavor! This cookie is a bit more delicate than some of the others in this book, so it won't stand tumbling about in travels, but it tastes so good, it's well worth making for the home cookie jar.

3½ cups Four Flour Bean Mix (pages 38–39)
1½ teaspoons xanthan gum
1 rounded teaspoon baking soda
½ teaspoon salt
1 cup margarine or butter
1 cup granulated sugar
1 cup brown sugar
1 egg
¾ cup vegetable oil
1 teaspoon vanilla
2 cups crushed GF cornflakes
1 cup almond slices, crushed (see Note)
⅔ cup coconut
½ cup chopped pecans

Preheat the oven to 325°.

In a medium bowl, combine the flour mix, xanthan gum, baking soda, and salt. Set aside.

In the bowl of your mixer, cream the margarine and sugars until light and fluffy. Add the egg and beat until well incorporated. Blend in the oil and vanilla. With a spoon, fold in the cornflakes, crushed almonds, coconut, and pecans.

Drop onto ungreased cookie sheets by teaspoonfuls, placing at least 1½ inches apart. Bake at 325° for 12 to 14 minutes. *Makes 6½ dozen cookies.*

Nutrients per cookie: Calories 100, Fat 6 g, Carbohydrate 10 g, Cholesterol 10 mg, Sodium 65 mg, Fiber 1 g, Protein 1 g

NOTE: To crush the almonds, place in a plastic bag and crush to oatmeal-size pieces with a rolling pin.

Chocolate Chip Cookies

350°

You don't have to miss these old favorites now that we can make them gluten free. This recipe may be halved to make 3 dozen cookies.

3¼ cups Four Flour Bean Mix (pages 38–39)
½ teaspoon xanthan gum
1 teaspoon baking soda
1 teaspoon salt
2 teaspoons Egg Replacer
1 cup (2 sticks) margarine or butter
1 cup brown sugar
½ cup granulated sugar
2 eggs
1 teaspoon vanilla
1½ cups chocolate chips
1 cup chopped walnuts or pecans (optional)

Preheat oven to 350°. Grease 2 cookie sheets.

In a medium bowl, whisk together the flour, xanthan gum, baking soda, salt, and Egg Replacer. Set aside.

In bowl of mixer, cream the margarine and sugars. Beat in the eggs and vanilla. With mixer on low, add the dry ingredients until just incorporated. Stir in the chocolate chips. Add nuts if using. Drop by teaspoonfuls onto prepared cookie sheets. Bake at 350° for 10 minutes. Remove from cookie sheets while still hot. *Makes 6 dozen cookies.*

Nutrients per cookie: Calories 80, Fat 4 g, Carbohydrate 11 g, Cholesterol 15 mg, Sodium 80 mg, Fiber 0, Protein 1 g

No-Bake Peanut Butter Bars

Easy enough even for children to make; a satisfying, chewy treat for the whole family.

6 cups gluten-free puffed or crisped rice cereal
1 cup raisins
1 cup dark corn syrup
1 cup chunky peanut butter
1 cup sugar

Butter a 9″ × 13″ oblong baking pan.

In a large bowl, mix the cereal and raisins together. Set aside. Heat the syrup, peanut butter, and sugar in a saucepan over low heat until it bubbles.

Pour the hot syrup over the rice cereal and raisins and blend together. Press the mixture into the prepared pan. Cut into squares when cool. *Makes 2 dozen 2 × 2-inch cookies.*

Nutrients per cookie: Calories 160, Fat 5 g, Carbohydrate 28 g, Cholesterol 0, Sodium 10 mg, Fiber 1 g, Protein 3 g

Butterscotch Brownies

350°

If you're hungry for the taste of cakelike brownies, these are my first choice, for they are easy to make and turn out moist and flavorful. They also will completely satisfy those who can eat gluten. The rice and soy flours may be replaced with 1½ cups Four-Flour Bean Mix.

½ cup (1 stick) margarine (see Note)
2 cups firmly packed brown sugar
1 teaspoon vanilla
3 eggs
1 cup rice flour
½ cup soy flour
2 teaspoons baking powder
½ teaspoon salt
1 cup finely chopped nuts

NOTE: For an even more tender bar, try Butter Flavor Crisco.

Cream margarine with the brown sugar. Add vanilla and eggs and beat with electric mixer until light. Combine the flours, baking powder, and salt. Add to egg mixture. Mix at low speed until blended. Stir in the nuts.

Spread the mixture evenly in a greased 9″ × 13″ pan. Bake in a preheated 350° oven for 25 to 30 minutes, or until top is light brown. Cool 10 to 15 minutes before cutting into bars. *Makes 2 dozen bars.*

Nutrients per cookie: Calories 150, Fat 8 g, Carbohydrate 20 g, Cholesterol 25 mg, Sodium 243 mg, Fiber 1 g, Protein 2 g

Chunky Chocolate Squares

350°

For all chocolate lovers. A no-fuss cookie, rich with nuts and chocolate.

2½ cups Four Flour Bean Mix (pages 38–39) or 1¼ cups rice flour and 1¼ cups soy flour
1 teaspoon xanthan gum
1½ teaspoons baking soda
½ teaspoon salt
¾ cup (1½ sticks) margarine or butter
1 cup brown sugar
¾ cup corn syrup
2 eggs
1 teaspoon vanilla
One 8-ounce package semisweet chocolate squares
1 cup chopped nuts

Preheat oven to 350°.

In a small bowl, combine the flour mix (or rice and soy flours), baking soda, and salt. Set aside. In the bowl of your mixer, beat butter and brown sugar with mixer at medium speed until fluffy. Slowly beat in the corn syrup, eggs, and vanilla. Beat in the prepared flour mixture until blended. Cut the chocolate squares into ½-inch chunks. Stir in the nuts and half the chocolate chunks.

Spread the batter evenly in an ungreased 15½″ × 10½″ jelly roll pan or a cookie sheet with raised sides. Sprinkle the remaining chocolate on top. Bake for 30 minutes or until lightly browned. Cool in pan before cutting into 2-inch squares. *Makes 3 dozen cookies.*

Nutrients per cookie: Calories 150, Fat 7 g, Carbohydrate 21 g, Cholesterol 20 mg, Sodium 130 mg, Fiber 1 g, Protein 2 g

Hello Dollys

325°

A rich candylike bar cookie with a combination of flavors that melts in your mouth. Extra easy to make.

½ cup (1 stick) margarine
1 cup crushed GF cereal (see Note)
1 cup shredded sweetened coconut
6 ounces (½ package) chocolate chips
6 ounces (½ package) butterscotch chips
1 can sweetened condensed milk
1 cup chopped nuts

Preheat oven to 325°.

In a 9″ × 13″ pan, melt the margarine. Add in layers the rest of the ingredients in the order listed. Bake for 30 minutes. When cool, cut in 1- to 1½-inch squares. *Makes 4½ to 5 dozen cookies.*

NOTE: Good also with dried GF bread crumbs with 1 tablespoon of sugar added. Absolutely wonderful with Ginger-Almond cookie crumbs.

Nutrients per cookie: Calories 160, Fat 9 g, Carbohydrate 21 g, Cholesterol 20 mg, Sodium 105 mg, Fiber 1 g, Protein 2 g

Orange-Slice Bars 350°

This recipe, clipped from a magazine over twenty-five years ago, became a family Christmas favorite. Even converted to the rice-soy flour mixture, it remains one. This cookie keeps and travels well.

NOTE: You may replace the rice and soy flours with the Four Flour Bean Mix.

1 pound candy orange slices
1½ cups rice flour
½ cup soy flour
1 teaspoon xanthan gum
½ teaspoon salt
3 cups light brown sugar
4 eggs, slightly beaten
1 cup chopped nuts
1 teaspoon vanilla

Cut orange slices into small pieces with scissors dipped in cold water (or in sugar). Add to flours and salt. Add remaining ingredients and mix well. Spread in greased 9″ × 13″ pan or two 8″ × 8″ pans. Bake in preheated 350° oven for about 45 minutes. Cool in pan. Cut into 1 × 2-inch bars. *Makes 3 to 4 dozen bars.*

Nutrients per cookie: Calories 110, Fat 2 g, Carbohydrate 23 g, Cholesterol 20 mg, Sodium 30 mg, Fiber 1 g, Protein 2 g

Orange Shortbread

300°

A very easy cookie and very satisfying. This is simply pressed into the pan and baked.

2¼ cups Four Flour Bean Mix (pages 38–39)
1 teaspoon xanthan gum
¼ teaspoon salt
Grated rind of 1 orange
1 cup (2 sticks) butter or margarine
½ cup sugar plus 2 tablespoons

Preheat oven to 300°.

In a medium bowl, whisk together the flour mix, xanthan gum, salt, and orange rind. Set aside.

In the bowl of your mixer, cream the butter and sugar. With the mixer on low, blend in the dry ingredients. (You may want to finish this by using your hands to blend.) Pat the dough into an 8″ × 12″ oblong pan and bake for 25 to 30 minutes. The top will brown only slightly. While still warm cut into 1 × 1½-inch cookies. *Makes about 2½ dozen cookies.*

Nutrients per cookie: Calories 190, Fat 11 g, Carbohydrate 24 g, Cholesterol 30 mg, Sodium 210 mg, Fiber 1 g, Protein 2 g

Fudge Brownies

350°

Use only one pan for mixing these easy chocolate treats. They really do taste like fudge and are so good no one will guess they're gluten free.

¾ cup Four Flour Bean Mix or GF Mix (pages 38–39)
½ (scant) teaspoon xanthan gum
1 teaspoon Egg Replacer
½ cup (1 stick) butter or margarine
2 squares unsweetened chocolate
1 cup sugar
2 eggs
1 teaspoon vanilla
½ cup chopped walnuts

Preheat oven to 350°. Grease an 8″ × 8″ square cake pan.

In a measuring cup, whisk the flour mix, xanthan gum, and Egg Replacer. Set aside.

In a medium saucepan, melt the butter and chocolate. Remove from heat and stir in sugar. Beat in the eggs, one at a time. Add the vanilla. Stir in the flour and nuts. Spoon into the prepared pan and bake for 30 minutes. Be careful not to overbake and dry out the cookies. Cool before cutting into 16 squares. *Makes 16 brownies.*

Nutrients per cookie: Calories 170, Fat 10 g, Carbohydrate 19 g, Cholesterol 40 mg, Sodium 70 mg, Fiber 1 g, Protein 2 g

Chewy Fruit Bars 350°

This moist, chewy bar keeps and travels well. It has a light fruitcake flavor, so is especially tasty for a Christmas cookie.

10 ounces fruit cake mix
½ cup fruit juice (orange, apple, or cranberry)
1 teaspoon grated orange peel
2 eggs
½ cup shortening
1⅓ cups brown sugar
¾ cup rice flour
¾ cup soy flour
1 teaspoon baking powder
1 teaspoon cinnamon
½ teaspoon salt

Preheat oven to 350°. Grease a 9″ × 13″ oblong pan or a cookie sheet with raised sides and dust with rice flour.

In a small bowl, combine the fruit cake mix, fruit juice, and grated orange peel. Set aside.

In a mixing bowl, beat together the eggs, shortening, and brown sugar. Combine the flours, baking powder, cinnamon, and salt and add to the egg-shortening mixture. Stir in the fruit mix.

Spread the dough in the prepared pan and bake for 25 to 30 minutes. Let cool slightly and cut into 2-inch squares or diamond shapes by marking diagonally across pan in both directions. *Makes 30 bars.*

Nutrients per cookie: Calories 90, Fat 4 g, Carbohydrate 11 g, Cholesterol 15 mg, Sodium 55 mg, Fiber 0, Protein 2 g

Shaped Cookies

Gingersnaps (Revised) 325°

For the nip and tingle of the old-fashioned gingersnap, try these cookies using the flavors of the new flours of bean and sorghum. There is no rolling out to these. Just roll them off the tip of the spoon, and they'll form the familiar round gingersnap shape as they bake.

4 cups Four Flour Bean Mix (pages 38–39)
1 teaspoon xanthan gum
3 teaspoons baking soda
2½ teaspoons ground ginger
1 teaspoon cinnamon
½ teaspoon ground cloves
¾ cup (1½ sticks) margarine or butter
2 cups sugar
2 eggs, well beaten
½ cup molasses
1 teaspoon vinegar

Preheat oven to 325°. Grease 2 cookie sheets.

In a medium bowl, whisk together the flour mix, xanthan gum, baking soda, ginger, cinnamon, and cloves. Set aside.

In the bowl of your mixer, cream the butter and sugar. Add the eggs and beat until smooth. Add the molasses and vinegar. Stir in the dry ingredients until well blended. The dough should be thick enough to form soft balls. If not, add more of the flour mix until the desired consistency is achieved.

Roll off from the tip of a teaspoon onto the cookie sheets a dough ball about the size of a walnut. Space about 1½ inches apart. Bake for about 12 minutes. *Makes about 10 dozen cookies.*

Nutrients per cookie: Calories 45, Fat 1½ g, Carbohydrate 8 g, Cholesterol 5 mg, Sodium 45 mg, Fiber 0, Protein 0

Old-fashioned Sugar Cookies (Revised) 350°

My first sugar cookies were so hard to handle that when I asked what recipes needed revision in this book, several celiacs shouted, "The sugar cookies." One admitted that she almost cried when they swelled and ran so you couldn't see the outlines. These are easier to handle and keep their shapes far better.

1 cup rice flour
¾ cup tapioca flour
¾ cup cornstarch
2½ teaspoons xanthan gum
1 teaspoon salt
1 cup sugar
1 cup shortening
1 egg or ¼ cup liquid egg substitute
2 teaspoons vanilla
¼ cup (or more) potato starch flour for kneading
Colored sugars, sprinkles, or frosting for decorating (optional)

Preheat oven to 350°.

In a small bowl, whisk together the flours, cornstarch, xanthan gum, and salt. Set aside.

In a mixing bowl, cream the sugar and shortening. Beat in the egg and vanilla. Add the dry ingredients, mixing enough to combine. The dough should form a soft ball. With your hands, knead in enough of the potato starch flour to make the dough easy to handle and roll out.

Working with half at a time, place a piece of plastic wrap over the ball and roll out to about ⅛ inch thickness. Cut into desired shapes and place on ungreased cookie sheet. Decorate with colored sugars before baking or use frosting to decorate after baking if desired. (With this dough you can use all the scraps. Just scrape them together and roll out again. They will not get tough.)

Bake for about 13 minutes. Cool very slightly before removing from cookie sheet. *Makes 3 dozen 2½-inch cookies.*

Nutrients per cookie: Calories 140, Fat 7 g, Carbohydrate 18 g, Cholesterol 5 mg, Sodium 75 mg, Fiber 0, Protein 1 g

Pralines

375°

A firm, flat cookie with a flavor reminiscent of the New Orleans candy from which it gets its name. This is another good traveler and keeper, for the flavor seems to improve with age.

½ cup (1 stick) butter or margarine
1½ cups dark brown sugar
2 eggs
¾ cup rice flour
¾ cup soy flour
½ cup chopped pecans

Grease two baking sheets.

In a mixing bowl, beat butter and sugar together until creamy. Beat in eggs and then flours. Add nuts. Chill 1 hour.

Roll pieces of dough into 1-inch balls. Place on prepared baking sheets 3 inches apart. Moisten bottom of glass tumbler; press balls to flatten to ⅛ inch thickness. Bake in preheated 375° oven 10 to 12 minutes, or until lightly browned. Remove immediately from baking sheets and cool. *Makes 3 dozen cookies.*

Nutrients per cookie: Calories 80, Fat 4 g, Carbohydrate 11 g, Cholesterol 10 mg, Sodium 45 mg, Fiber 0, Protein 1 g

Refrigerator Roll (Revised)

375°

Make up this basic dough and add your choice of nuts, raisins, coconut, candied cherries, or chocolate. Freeze it and then take out to bake when you feel like having cookies.

1½ cups Four Flour Bean Mix or GF Mix (pages 38–39)
¾ teaspoon xanthan gum
1 teaspoon baking powder
½ cup (1 stick) margarine or butter
1¼ cups sugar
1 egg
1 teaspoon vanilla

ADDITION:
½ to 1 cup chopped nuts
½ cup chopped raisins
½ to ¾ cup shredded coconut, chopped candied cherries, or citron
or 1 or 2 squares melted chocolate

In a medium bowl, whisk together the flour, xanthan gum, and baking powder. Set aside.

Cream the butter and sugar. Beat in the egg and vanilla. Add the dry ingredients. The dough should be similar to pastry. Add one of the additions.

For a marbled look to the chocolate, use less of the melted chocolate and just blend until you achieve a marbled texture. For a butterscotch flavor, use dark brown sugar. You may separate the dough and make two different kinds of cookies from the one batch.

If the dough is not stiff enough to form a ball, add flour 1 tablespoon at a time until the right texture is reached. Roll the dough in a long roll about 1½ inches in diameter and 12 inches long, or into two shorter rolls, each about 6 inches long. Wrap in plastic wrap and refrigerate 1 hour before slicing about ⅙ inch thick. Bake on greased cookie sheets in preheated 375° oven for 10 to 12 minutes. *Makes about 6 dozen cookies.*

Nutrients per cookie: Calories 30, Fat 5 g, Carbohydrate 6 g, Cholesterol 5 mg, Sodium 15 mg, Fiber 0, Protein 0

Jam-Filled Crunchies

350°

A rich, tasty cookie for special treats. The surprise is in the crunch. These are tender and do not travel well.

1 cup (2 sticks) butter or margarine
⅔ cup sugar
1 teaspoon vanilla
1 egg
1½ cups rice flour
½ cup soy flour
¾ cup crushed potato chips
½ cup chopped pecans
¼ cup raspberry or apricot jam

Preheat oven to 350°.

In a mixing bowl, beat butter, all but 2 tablespoons of sugar, and vanilla until fluffy. Stir in the egg, flours, potato chips, and pecans. Mix until blended.

Roll dough into 1¼-inch balls. Place on ungreased cookie sheets and flatten each ball with the back of a teaspoon dipped in the remaining sugar. Dot each cookie center with ¼ teaspoon jam.

Bake for 16 to 18 minutes, or until lightly browned. These should be stored airtight for a couple of days or frozen. *Makes 3½ dozen cookies.*

Nutrients per cookie: Calories 90, Fat 6 g, Carbohydrate 10 g, Cholesterol 15 mg, Sodium 60 mg, Fiber 0, Protein 1 g

Ginger-Almond Sticks

350°

A crisp, spicy biscotti to go with your coffee, milk, or wine. This very different cookie is baked twice, but after you've tasted one you'll agree they're well worth the extra trouble.

1 cup slivered almonds
¾ cup sugar
½ cup (1 stick) butter or margarine
½ cup molasses
¼ cup grated fresh ginger
4 eggs
3 cups GF Mix or Four Flour Bean Mix (pages 38–39)
1 tablespoon baking powder
1 tablespoon cinnamon
1 teaspoon nutmeg
½ teaspoon cloves
½ teaspoon allspice
1½ teaspoons xanthan gum

Preheat oven to 350°. Grease two cookie sheets.

Place almonds in an 8″ square pan and bake until lightly toasted, 10 to 15 minutes. Let cool and then chop coarsely and set aside.

In the bowl of your mixer, beat sugar, butter, molasses, and ginger until smooth. Add the eggs, one at a time, beating after each addition. Mix together the flour, baking powder, cinnamon, nutmeg, cloves, allspice, almonds, and xanthan gum. Add to the egg mixture, stirring to blend.

Using your hands, pat the dough into 4 flat loaves on the cookie sheets. Each loaf should be about ½ inch thick, 2 inches wide, and the length of the baking sheet. (I use plastic wrap to cover my hands as I pat the dough into shape.) Bake about 25 minutes, reversing the position of the cookie sheets in the oven halfway through the baking. When done, the loaves should be browned at the edges and springy to the touch.

Let loaves stand on the cookie sheets until cool, then cut into ½-inch-thick diagonal slices. Arrange the slices on their sides on the baking sheets and return to the oven to bake again until the cookies are brown and crisp, 15 to 18 minutes. Again, reverse the position of the baking sheets halfway through baking.

Let sticks cool to serve or store airtight up to 1 month, or freeze them. *Makes about 4 dozen sticks.*

NOTE: Be sure to save any broken sticks and all the crumbs. On page 149 there's a recipe for using the crumbs and leftovers for a pastry crust. A gourmet treat!

Nutrients per cookie: Calories 90, Fat 4 g, Carbohydrate 14 g, Cholesterol 25 mg, Sodium 50 mg, Fiber 0, Protein 1 g

Date Roll-ups

375°

This unusual cookie made of pastry wrapped around dates or nuts gives variety to a plate of mixed goodies. The tender cream cheese crust lends a different taste for the palate.

One 8-ounce package cream cheese
1 cup (2 sticks) butter or margarine
½ cup rice flour
½ cup tapioca flour
1 rounded teaspoon potato flour
½ cup cornstarch
1 teaspoon xanthan gum
1 teaspoon salt
One 12-ounce package pitted dates, or 1 cup walnut halves

Soften the cream cheese and cream it with the butter. Thoroughly blend the flours, cornstarch, xanthan gum, and salt. Add to the creamed mixture. This should resemble soft pie dough. Refrigerate for 1 hour or until firm.

Preheat oven to 375°.

Remove dough from refrigerator and work into two balls. Roll them out, one at a time, on a board sprinkled with powdered sugar. Cut with a pastry wheel into 1 × 4-inch oblongs. Roll these around the dates or walnuts.

Tuck the flap sides down and bake on cookie sheets for 15 or 20 minutes. *Makes approximately 6 dozen pastries.*

Nutrients per cookie: Calories 110, Fat 9 g, Carbohydrate 7 g, Cholesterol 20 mg, Sodium 130 mg, Fiber 0, Protein 2 g

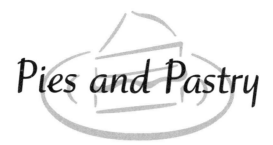

Pies and Pastry

Pastry and Crusts

Refrigerator Pies and Meringue-Topped Pies

Baked Pies

See Also

You don't have to give up pies on a wheat- or gluten-free diet. The fruit or cream fillings for many pies are gluten free. There are many recipes we can find in our old cookbooks, but the catch is the pastry. Every recipe calls for pastry flour, which means wheat.

Working with rice flour may be more difficult than wheat flour, but not impossible. And it makes a delicious pastry. With the addition of bean flours to our cooking we can make a wonderfully tasty crust using the Four Flour Bean Mix (pages 38–39). I've also suggested other easier ones such as cereal or crumb crusts. In addition, I've included a few of my favorite pie recipes, but in most cases you can use your own recipes for fruit pies as long as you remember to thicken with tapioca, rice flour, or cornstarch. These are listed under Fruit Fancies (page 161). If you see a cream pie recipe you think sounds good, check to see if it is thickened with egg yolks and/or cornstarch rather than wheat flour.

There are also many packaged pudding and pie fillings that are gluten free. Be sure to read the ingredient list on the box each time, for manufacturers do change formulas, and one that is safe for you one day may include wheat starch the next time you buy it.

Vinegar Pastry (Revised)

450°

Just before I was diagnosed, my aunt, a fine pastry maker, gave me all her secrets to making pastry. But it was all for naught when I started to experiment with rice flour. At first I used it alone in crusts, which fell apart on touching. With the new added tapioca and cornstarch, this crust handles much like our old wheat ones.

1 cup white rice flour
¾ cup tapioca flour
¾ cup cornstarch
1 rounded teaspoon xanthan gum
¾ teaspoon salt
1 tablespoon sugar
¾ cup shortening
1 egg, lightly beaten
1 tablespoon vinegar
2 to 3 tablespoons ice water

In a medium bowl, whisk together the flours, cornstarch, xanthan gum, salt, and sugar. Cut in the shortening. Blend together the beaten egg, vinegar, and cold water. Stir into the flour mixture, holding back some, until the pastry holds together and forms a ball. (Kneading will not toughen this pastry.)

Form two balls and place in a bowl; cover and refrigerate for 30 minutes. Remove and roll one ball at a time between 2 sheets of plastic wrap that have been dusted with sweet rice flour. To place in a pie tin: Remove top sheet and, using the other for ease of handling, invert the dough and drop it into the pan. Shape it into the curves before removing the second piece of plastic wrap. For a crust to be used later, bake in a preheated 450° oven for 10 to 12 minutes. For a filled pie, follow directions for that pie. *Makes two 9" crusts or a double-crusted pie.*

Nutrients per serving: Calories 170, Fat 90 g, Carbohydrate 19 g, Cholesterol 15 mg, Sodium 105 mg, Fiber 0, Protein 1 g

Four Flour Pastry

425°

Don't be afraid to try this pastry: It handles like wheat and is just as light and flaky. It's easy to mix and takes handling well.

2 cups Four Flour Bean Mix (pages 38–39)
¼ cup sweet rice flour
1 teaspoon xanthan gum
1 teaspoon baking powder
½ teaspoon salt
2 teaspoons sugar
⅓ cup margarine or butter
⅓ cup Butter Flavor Crisco
3 tablespoons liquid egg substitute or 1 small egg
1 tablespoon vinegar
3 tablespoons ice water
Sweet rice flour for rolling

In a medium bowl, whisk together the flours, xanthan gum, baking powder, salt, and sugar. Cut in the margarine and Crisco in small pieces until you have shortening the size of lima beans (not cornmeal).

Beat the egg with a fork and add the vinegar and ice water. Stir into the dry ingredients, forming a ball. You may refrigerate to chill, but it is not necessary.

Divide dough into two halves and roll the first half out onto plastic wrap dusted with sweet rice flour. Transfer to a pie tin by inverting the plastic wrap. Add the pie filling and roll out the second half of the dough. Place the second crust over the filling, seal the edges, and bake as directed for the filling used.

For a baked pie shell, prick the pastry with a fork on the sides and bottom. Bake in a preheated 425° oven for about 12 to 14 minutes. Cool before filling. *Makes one 2-crust pie or 2 pie shells.*

Nutrients per serving: Calories 185, Fat 85 g, Carbohydrate 26 g, Cholesterol 0, Sodium 105 mg, Fiber 1 g, Protein 1 g

Crumb Crust

A good use for the crumbs from your baking mistakes. Dry GF bread, cake, or cookie pieces in a 200° oven until crisp and dry, 1 or 2 hours. Then pulverize in a food processor. Store in your freezer to pull out when needed. The following recipe makes enough dough for a 10" springform pan or to line an 8" pie pan. Increase all measurements slightly for a deep 9" pie tin.

1½ cups GF crumbs
1 tablespoon sugar
1 teaspoon cinnamon
¼ cup melted butter or margarine

Put all the ingredients in a 1-gallon plastic food storage bag. Shake together to mix. Press the dough evenly onto the bottom and sides of the greased pie pan or the bottom of the springform pan.

If the pie is to be baked, fill before baking. If the pie filling is already cooked (cream pie, lemon, package mix, and so on), then bake your crust in preheated 400° oven for about 8 minutes before filling.

Nutrients per serving: Calories 130, Fat 5 g, Carbohydrate 19 g, Cholesterol 12 mg, Sodium 133 mg, Fiber 1 g, Protein 2 g

Cereal Crust

Probably the easiest of all crusts. I make this crust in the same plastic bag in which I crush the cereal, thus eliminating one bowl to wash.

2 cups GF cereal
3 tablespoons melted butter or margarine
2 tablespoons sugar

Crush the cereal in a plastic bag, then add the butter and sugar and shake together. Pat the mixture into a 9″ pie tin. If the pie is to be baked, pour the mixture into the unbaked cereal crust and bake according to the filling recipe. If the pie filling is already cooked, bake the crust in preheated 400° oven for about 6 minutes before filling it. Cool before serving.

Nutrients per serving: Calories 80, Fat 4 g, Carbohydrate 10 g, Cholesterol 10 mg, Sodium 110 mg, Fiber 0, Protein 1 g

Ginger Cookie Crust

On page 139, you'll find a recipe for Ginger-Almond Sticks. If you have any crumbs or broken pieces from this recipe, save them for this crust for a truly gourmet pie or cheesecake. It's worth making the cookies just for the crumbs. Make and bake a whole recipe and store the crumbs for crusts.

For a 9″ pie you'll need 1½ cups of crumbs and 2½ tablespoons of melted margarine or butter, a little less of each for an 8″ pie. If you are short of crumbs, you can use ½ cup crushed cornflakes to make up the difference.

Nutrients per serving: Calories 180, Fat 9 g, Carbohydrate 22 g, Cholesterol 45 mg, Sodium 115 mg, Fiber 1 g, Protein 2 g

Meringue Shell

275°

A sweet, frothy shell for light, fluffy pies.

- 2 egg whites
- ¼ teaspoon cream of tartar
- ¼ teaspoon salt
- ½ teaspoon vanilla
- ½ cup sugar

Place the egg whites, cream of tartar, salt, and vanilla in a mixing bowl and beat with an electric mixer until foamy. Beating constantly, add the sugar about 1 tablespoon at a time. Continue beating until very stiff and glossy. Grease a deep 9″ pie pan and spread the mixture on the sides and bottom. Bake in a preheated 275° oven for 1 hour. Cool away from drafts before filling.

Nutrients per serving: Calories 43, Fat 0, Carbohydrate 101 g, Cholesterol 0, Sodium 65 mg, Fiber 0, Protein 7 g

Refrigerator Pies and Meringue-Topped Pies

Angel Pie (Pineapple)

A melt-in-your-mouth dessert.

- Meringue Shell, see above
- ¾ cup sugar
- ¼ cup cornstarch
- ½ teaspoon salt
- One 20-ounce can crushed pineapple
- 2 tablespoons lemon juice
- 2 tablespoons butter or margarine
- 2 egg yolks, slightly beaten
- 1 cup whipping cream or 2 cups nondairy whipped topping

Prepare and bake the meringue shell.

Combine sugar, cornstarch, and salt in a saucepan. Gradually stir in the pineapple and its juice, lemon juice, and butter. Cook over medium heat, stirring constantly, until thickened. Gradually add a little of the hot pineapple to the egg yolks, then combine this mixture with the hot mixture in the saucepan.

Cook 1 or 2 minutes more, stirring constantly. Chill until cold. Whip the cream and fold into the pineapple mixture. Pour into the meringue shell. Refrigerate until serving time. *Makes 6 servings.*

VARIATIONS: Substitute one 12-ounce carton Cranberry Orange Sauce plus ⅓ cup orange juice for the pineapple.

Substitute one 17-ounce can apricot halves, drained and puréed, plus ⅓ cup reserved drained juice.

Nutrients per serving: Calories 350, Fat 18 g, Carbohydrate 47 g, Cholesterol 125 mg, Sodium 270 mg, Fiber 1 g, Protein 2 g

Basic Cream Pie Filling (Revised)

This filling can be as rich as you choose by changing the milk to part cream or to all cream. Use it with bananas, pineapple, or with GF canned fruit pie fillings. Prepare the desired single crust for a 9" pie (cereal, crumb, or vinegar pastry) and bake according to the recipe. Then make the filling. Use the following or the easy microwave recipe on page 152.

½ cup sugar
¼ cup cornstarch
2½ cups 4% milk or nondairy liquid
Pinch salt
3 egg yolks
1 tablespoon vanilla

In a medium saucepan, whisk together the sugar and cornstarch. Whisk in the milk and add the salt. Bring to a boil over moderately high heat, whisking constantly. Lower the heat to medium and cook, whisking constantly, for 2 minutes, or until the mixture is thickened.

In a small bowl, whisk the egg yolks until well blended. Add a little of the hot mixture to the yolks and slowly blend. Return the mixture to the saucepan. Cook 2 minutes more, whisking constantly. Remove from the heat and stir in the vanilla. *Makes 8 servings as a custard.*

Follow the directions below for your favorite pie.

BANANA CREAM PIE: Line the baked pie shell with 2 bananas cut into ¼-inch slices. Pour the cream filling over the bananas. Chill and decorate with whipped cream fluted around the edges before serving. *Makes 6 servings.*

PINEAPPLE CREAM PIE: Add an 8-ounce can crushed pineapple, drained, to the cream filling before pouring into the baked pie shell. Chill and decorate as above with whipped cream at edges. *Makes 6 servings.*

COCONUT CREAM PIE: Add 1 cup sweetened flaked coconut to the pie filling while it is still hot. Pour into the baked shell. Top with a meringue of 2 egg whites beaten stiff with 2 tablespoons sugar. Drizzle on a couple of tablespoons of coconut. Bake in preheated 425° oven until the meringue browns. Watch carefully; don't let the meringue get too dark. *Makes 6 to 8 servings.*

Nutrients per serving: Calories 350, Fat 14 g, Carbohydrate 48 g, Cholesterol 220 mg, Sodium 210 mg, Fiber 0, Protein 8 g

Microwave Cream Pie Filling

This is so easy, you may never stir up a custard sauce over the stove again. The recipe calls for milk, but I prefer to use part cream or some evaporated milk for a richer custard. For the nondairy liquid I use a coffee creamer and thin it with a little water.

⅓ cup sugar (or to taste)	**2 cups milk or nondairy liquid**
¼ cup cornstarch	**2 egg yolks**
⅛ teaspoon salt	**1½ teaspoons vanilla**

In a 4-cup glass measure or bowl, combine the sugar, cornstarch, and salt. Add about ¼ cup of milk and stir until cornstarch is dissolved. Add the remaining milk and whisk until smooth. Cover with wax paper and cook on High in the microwave for 5 to 7 minutes, stirring twice while the mixture comes to a boil and thickens. Whisk until smooth.

In a small bowl, beat the egg yolks lightly. Whisk in about ½ cup of the hot mixture. Stir this into the remaining milk mixture, return to the microwave, and cook, uncovered, for 1 minute on High. Blend in the vanilla. *Makes 2¼ cups, or 6 servings.*

Nutrients per serving: Calories 310, Fat 4 g, Carbohydrate 37 g, Cholesterol 80 mg, Sodium 230 mg, Fiber 0, Protein 5 g

Easy Lemon Pie

350°

A tart and tangy lemon pie that can be stirred up with very little fuss or bother. This takes no stovetop cooking before pouring into an unbaked pie shell and letting the oven do the work.

One unbaked (9-inch) piecrust	**⅓ cup plus 2 tablespoons lemon juice**
3 eggs, separated	**¼ cup butter or margarine, melted**
1¼ cups sugar	
Zest of one lemon	

Preheat oven to 350°.

Place egg whites in the bowl of your mixer. Beat until the eggs form soft peaks. Remove to another bowl.

In the same bowl, beat the egg yolks, sugar, lemon zest, and lemon juice for 3 minutes or until smooth. Add the butter and blend. Gently fold in the beaten whites and pour into the prepared crust. Bake for 30 to 35 minutes. *Makes 6 servings.*

Nutrients per serving: Calories 300, Fat 10 g, Carbohydrate 50 g, Cholesterol 100 mg, Sodium 120 mg, Fiber 0, Protein 4 g

Boston Cream Pie

Now this cake-pie combination is not forbidden fruit for the gluten intolerant.

1 recipe Classic Sponge Cake, page 94
½ recipe Basic Cream Pie Filling, page 151
One 27-ounce can GF prepared fruit pie filling (cherry, berry, apple, or other)
Whipped cream topping or a nondairy substitute

Prepare the sponge cake recipe and bake it in two 8″ round cake pans. They will take about 10 to 15 minutes less time to bake than in a tube pan. Remove from pans to cool on wire racks.

Spread one layer with the cream pie filling. Top with the second cake layer and top this with the prepared fruit pie filling. Make a decorative edge around the outside of the top with whipped cream or nondairy topping. Refrigerate.

Cut into wedges to serve. This is a rich pie and can easily be cut to serve 12.

NOTE: Instead of canned pie filling, you may use fresh fruit, cooked and sweetened to taste and thickened with 1 to 2 tablespoons sweet rice flour. You will need 1½ to 2 cups fruit filling.

Nutrients per serving: Calories 310, Fat 11 g, Carbohydrate 47 g, Cholesterol 175 mg, Sodium 170 mg, Fiber 0, Protein 6 g

Raisin–Sour Cream Pie 450°/325°

An old favorite that's quick to make; it will disappear just as fast. You may use a regular pastry crust or cereal or crumb crust for this pie. If you use a cereal crust, you might like to add 1 teaspoon of cinnamon to the cereal before crushing. Prepare the crust but don't bake it. Prepare the following filling:

3 eggs
1¼ cups sugar
¼ teaspoon salt
1 teaspoon cinnamon
¼ teaspoon cloves
1½ cups sour cream or nondairy substitute
1½ cups seedless raisins

Preheat oven to 450°.

Beat together eggs, sugar, salt, cinnamon, and cloves. Blend in the sour cream or nondairy substitute. Stir in the raisins.

Pour into a pastry-lined 9″ pie pan. Bake at 450° for 10 minutes, then turn to 325° for 20 to 25 minutes, or until a knife inserted in the center comes out clean. Serve slightly warm or cold. Refrigerate if kept more than several hours after baking. *Makes 6 to 8 servings.*

Nutrients per serving: Calories 330, Fat 12 g, Carbohydrate 56 g, Cholesterol 100 mg, Sodium 130 mg, Fiber 1 g, Protein 5 g

Apple Pear Deluxe Pie 400°

You can use any of your favorite recipes for regular apple pie, but this will be a change for the palate.

Vinegar Pastry (Revised) (page 146)
4 cups peeled, diced tart apples
1 cup plus ½ teaspoon sugar
2 tablespoons tapioca flour
⅛ teaspoon salt
½ teaspoon cinnamon
4 canned pear halves
2 tablespoons rum
2 tablespoons butter or margarine
1 tablespoon milk

Preheat oven to 400°.

Prepare pastry and fit half into a 9″ pie pan.

Place apples in a large mixing bowl. Mix 1 cup sugar, tapioca flour, salt, and cinnamon, and add to the apples, tumbling to coat thoroughly. Set aside.

Crush the pears and spread the pulp in the bottom of your pastry-lined pan. Sprinkle with rum. Pour the apple mixture over the pears and dot with butter. Add the top crust, seal, and crimp edges. Cut slits for vents. Brush the top of the pastry with milk and sprinkle on about ½ teaspoon sugar. Bake in 400° oven for 45 minutes, or until the apples are tender. Serve warm. *Makes 8 servings.*

Nutrients per serving: Calories 360, Fat 13 g, Carbohydrate 60 g, Cholesterol 20 mg, Sodium 170 mg, Fiber 2 g, Protein 1 g

Pecan Pie 350°

A southern favorite—easy to make, high in calories. Serve small portions, for this is a rich pie. The texture of a cereal crust goes well with this. If you use it, try chopping a couple of tablespoons of the nuts very fine and adding them to the crust mixture before patting into the pie pan.

3 eggs
1 cup dark corn syrup
1 cup brown sugar
1 teaspoon vanilla
2 tablespoons margarine, melted
1½ cups pecan bits or halves

Preheat oven to 350°.

In a mixing bowl, beat the eggs. Add the corn syrup, sugar, vanilla, and melted margarine. Stir together until blended. Fold in the pecans. Pour into an unbaked pie shell and bake for 50 to 55 minutes, until a knife inserted near the center comes out clean. Cool before serving. *Makes a large 9" pie that can serve 8 to 10.*

Nutrients per serving: Calories 290, Fat 14 g, Carbohydrate 43 g, Cholesterol 20 mg, Sodium 75 mg, Fiber 1 g, Protein 2 g

Rum Pecan Pie 425°

Rum gives a new taste to the preceding pie. Prepare an unbaked crust, either the cereal or crumb crust, omitting the sugar.

2 eggs
⅔ cup brown sugar
⅔ cup dark corn syrup
⅓ cup dark rum
2 tablespoons butter or margarine, melted
1 teaspoon vanilla
2 cups broken pecans

Preheat oven to 425°.

Break eggs into a mixing bowl. Beat slightly. Add the rest of the ingredients except the nuts. Beat until well blended. Then fold in the nuts. Pour into the unbaked pie shell and bake at 425° for 45 to 50 minutes. *Makes 8 to 10 servings.*

Nutrients per serving: Calories 530, Fat 29 g, Carbohydrate 60 g, Cholesterol 75 mg, Sodium 240 mg, Fiber 3 g, Protein 6 g

Tropical Tofu Pie

350°

The blend of several tropical fruit flavors plus the tofu makes this a welcome dessert that is not too sweet. It tastes a bit like a light cheesecake. This is served cold, so it can be made ahead. Prepare a deep 9" cereal or crumb crust, using ½ teaspoon cinnamon for added flavor if desired. Do not bake the crust.

One 14-ounce block firm or medium tofu
3 eggs
⅔ cup sugar
2 teaspoons grated orange peel
2 tablespoons lemon juice
2 ripe bananas
One 8-ounce can crushed pineapple

Preheat oven to 350°.

Place the tofu, broken into chunks, in a food processor. Process lightly. Add eggs, sugar, orange peel, and lemon juice. Process until well mixed. Add the bananas, cut into chunks, and process until smooth. Stir in the well-drained crushed pineapple. Pour into the prepared crust.

Bake for about 45 to 50 minutes, or until center is firm. Cool. Refrigerate until served. The pie may be served plain or with whipped cream or crushed fruit as topping. *Makes 8 to 10 servings.*

Nutrients per serving: Calories 170, Fat 6 g, Carbohydrate 25 g, Cholesterol 65 mg, Sodium 35 mg, Fiber 1 g, Protein 9 g

Lemon Sponge Pie

350°

A very different lemon pie with a delightful tart taste, this is simple to make but turns out layered with a frothy, creamy top.

Vinegar Pastry (Revised) (page 146)
3 eggs
3 tablespoons butter or margarine
¾ cup sugar
2 tablespoons sweet rice flour
¼ teaspoon salt
1½ cups buttermilk
3 tablespoons lemon juice

Preheat oven to 350°.

Prepare pastry and use half to line a 9″ pie shell, reserving remaining pastry for another use.

Separate the eggs, putting the yolks in a large mixing bowl and the whites in a small one. Melt the butter and set aside. Beat the yolks with an electric mixer and add ½ cup of the sugar, rice flour, and salt. Stir in the melted butter, buttermilk, and lemon juice.

Beat the egg whites until they form peaks and gradually beat in the remaining ¼ cup sugar. Fold these into the yolk mix. Pour into the prepared pie shell. Bake in 350° oven for 20 to 25 minutes, or until a knife inserted in center comes out clean. *Makes 6 to 8 servings.*

Nutrients per serving: Calories 180, Fat 8 g, Carbohydrate 24 g, Cholesterol 195 mg, Sodium 230 mg, Fiber 0, Protein 5 g

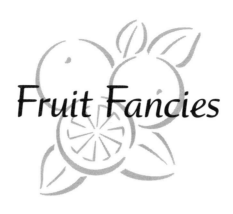

Fruit Fancies

See Also

Plain fruits, either fresh or canned, are among the few desserts one can safely order out on a gluten-free diet. We pick them from the buffet trays and notice them on any menu. But fruits in any baked form in a restaurant or at a friend's house have to be suspect.

Here I've put together a small collection of ways of using fresh, canned, or frozen fruit in baking for brunch, lunch, or dinner. Some of them are old familiars with a change to our gluten-free flours. Others may be new to you. All are enthusiastically endorsed by friends who don't have to stick to any diet.

Fruit-Filled Meringues

275°

When a friend called desperately about a dinner party she was hosting and asked, "Have you any suggestions for dessert you can eat? I don't have any of your flour to bake with," I replied, "Why not meringues? They don't take flour."

It's a good answer, but don't leave them for someone else to try. Meringues are very simple to make and can be made several days ahead and stored in a closed container. All you need are:

3 egg whites
¼ teaspoon cream of tartar
¾ cup sugar
Fresh or frozen berries for filling

In a metal or glass bowl, beat egg whites and cream of tartar until frothy. Gradually beat in the sugar, a little at a time, until mixture is very stiff and glossy.

Drop by spoonfuls in 3½-inch circles 1½ inches thick on brown paper on a baking sheet. With the back of a spoon make an indentation on each meringue. Bake in preheated 275° oven for about 1 hour. Turn oven off and leave the meringues in until oven has cooled.

To serve, fill with fresh or frozen and thawed berries and, if desired, top with whipped cream. *Makes 6 meringues.*

Nutrients per serving: Calories 60, Fat 0, Carbohydrate 13 g, Cholesterol 0, Sodium 30 mg, Fiber 2 g, Protein 2 g

Hawaiian Delight Meringues

400°

A fancy-looking dessert that takes but minutes of the cook's time.

One 30-ounce can pineapple slices
2 bananas
1 tablespoon lemon juice
3 tablespoons plus ½ cup sugar
½ teaspoon cinnamon
4 egg whites
¼ teaspoon cream of tartar

Drain the pineapple slices and arrange in a large buttered baking dish or on a buttered cookie sheet. Cut each banana into 5 pieces and place one piece on each slice of pineapple. Sprinkle with lemon juice.

Mix the 3 tablespoons of sugar with the cinnamon and sprinkle half of this over the fruits.

Beat the egg whites with the cream of tartar until soft peaks form. Add the rest of the sugar (reserving 1 tablespoon) a couple of tablespoons at a time, beating well after each addition. Beat until the whites form stiff peaks.

Spread the meringue over pineapple and bananas, using a swirling design. Sprinkle the remaining sugar over the meringues and bake in a preheated 400° oven for 10 minutes, or until the meringue is brown. Serve warm or cold.

If you are using fresh pineapple, peel, core, and cut into 10 slices. The pineapple does not need to be precooked. *Makes 8 to 10 servings.*

Nutrients per serving: Calories 140, Fat 0.5 g, Carbohydrate 33 g, Cholesterol 0, Sodium 25 mg, Fiber 2 g, Protein 2 g

Bavarian Cream with Fruit

This can be a glamorous-looking dessert, and by cutting out the high-fat creams usually used, the calories can be lowered considerably to fit in with today's fight against fat. This recipe includes changes for the lactose intolerant.

1 cup low-fat milk or nondairy substitute
1 envelope unflavored gelatin
2 tablespoons water
½ cup sugar
1 cup light sour cream or nondairy substitute
1 teaspoon almond flavoring for peaches or ½ teaspoon for berries
½ cup crushed fresh peaches, strawberries, or raspberries
1½ tablespoons sugar (or to taste)

In a medium saucepan, heat milk over medium heat, stirring frequently, until it just comes to a boil.

In a small bowl, soften gelatin in the water. Add the gelatin and ½ cup sugar to the milk. Cool to room temperature.

Whisk in the sour cream and almond flavoring. Add the 1½ tablespoons sugar to the fruit and stir in. Pour into a 1-quart mold. Cover and refrigerate until set. To serve, unmold onto a large plate or into a low serving bowl if using as a buffet dessert. If making single servings, spoon into parfait or dessert dishes. If desired, top with more of the fresh fruit or with a dab of whipped cream or nondairy topping and a piece of fruit or a sprig of mint. *Makes 6 to 8 servings.*

Nutrients per serving: Calories 135, Fat 2 g, Carbohydrate 27 g, Cholesterol 6 mg, Sodium 46 mg, Fiber 1 g, Protein 4 g

Peach Custard Pie   375°

An easy to make custard and fruit pie in a crisp, buttery crust. A summertime favorite when peaches are ripe. Also great with an apple filling rather than the peach.

1½ cups GF cereal
2 tablespoons sugar
3 tablespoons butter or margarine
3 medium-sized peaches
1 tablespoon lemon juice
½ teaspoon cinnamon
½ cup brown sugar, packed
2 eggs
1 cup sour cream or nondairy substitute

Crush the cereal in a plastic bag and add the sugar. Melt the butter, pour into bag, and mix. Pat into deep 9″ pie plate.

Slice the peaches into a bowl. Add lemon juice, cinnamon, and brown sugar, reserving 1 tablespoonful of sugar. Toss lightly and place on the cereal crust. Bake in preheated 375° oven for 15 minutes.

While this is baking, beat the eggs and add the sour cream and the remaining tablespoon of brown sugar. Pour this over the partly baked peaches and return to the oven for 20 to 25 minutes, until the custard jiggles very slightly.

Serve warm or cool. Will keep, covered with plastic wrap, in refrigerator for up to 2 days. *Makes 6 to 8 servings.*

For apple filling, put apple, lemon juice, spice, and sugar mixture in microwave for 3 minutes before pouring into cereal crust and baking. In the oven it takes a bit longer to bake before pouring on the custard topping.

Nutrients per serving: Calories 220, Fat 12 g, Carbohydrate 27 g, Cholesterol 80 mg, Sodium 135 mg, Fiber 1 g, Protein 3 g

Deep-dish Berry Pie with a Cream Cheese Crust

350°

A real crowd pleaser that is also good with other juicy fruits like peaches and plums. The recipe is given for an 8″ × 8″ baking dish but can be doubled for a 9″ × 13″ pan.

FILLING

5½ cups berries (blueberries, blackberries, raspberries, boysenberries, loganberries, or other)
1 cup sugar (or to taste)
3 tablespoons tapioca flour

CRUST

One 3-ounce package cream cheese
2 tablespoons butter or margarine
2 teaspoons sugar
¾ cup GF Mix (page 38)

Wash and drain berries. Pour about one-fourth of them into an 8″ × 8″ pan and mash. Toss the remaining whole berries with sugar and flour and add to pan. Set aside while making the crust.

Put cream cheese, butter, and sugar into a mixing bowl and beat with an electric mixer until well blended. Add the flour and mix again until blended. Roll dough into a ball and refrigerate until firm enough to roll easily, about 30 minutes.

Place the chilled pastry on plastic wrap, cover with another piece of plastic wrap, and roll until slightly larger than the pan. Remove top plastic and turn the pastry over onto the berries before removing the other plastic. (This makes for easy handling.) Tuck the crust overlap down the sides of the pan into your berries. Bake in preheated 350° oven for approximately 1 to 1¼ hours. *Makes 6 servings.*

Nutrients per serving: Calories 350, Fat 7 g, Carbohydrate 71 g, Cholesterol 20 mg, Sodium 60 mg, Fiber 5 g, Protein 3 g

Apple Pie with Streusel Topping 400°

An easy and delicious apple pie you can feed to anyone and expect raves. Use the Vinegar Pastry (Revised) (page 146) and show your friends how good gluten free can be.

One 9″ unbaked pastry crust
5 to 6 cups apple slices
3 tablespoons lemon juice
¼ cup GF Mix (page 38)
1 cup sugar
1 teaspoon cinnamon
¼ teaspoon nutmeg
½ cup chopped walnuts
½ cup raisins

STREUSEL
⅓ cup brown sugar
⅓ cup GF Mix
3 tablespoons butter or margarine

In a large bowl, toss apple slices with the lemon juice. Combine the flour mix, sugar, cinnamon, and nutmeg and toss again. Stir in the walnuts and raisins. Place in the unbaked crust and mix streusel by combining the brown sugar and flour mix. With your fingers or a fork, cut in the butter. Sprinkle evenly over the apples, covering them lightly. Bake at 400° for 50 minutes to 1 hour. Serve warm or cold. *Makes 6 servings.*

Nutrients per serving: Calories 610, Fat 20 g, Carbohydrate 108 g, Cholesterol 15 mg, Sodium 220 mg, Fiber 5 g, Protein 5 g

Pear Torte 375°

This is another fruit and custard baked in a crust, but a bit more elegant than the peach custard pie. Pears are often overlooked in baking by cooks more familiar with apples or berries, but this treat will show they shouldn't be.

CRUST

½ cup (1 stick) butter or margarine
⅓ cup sugar
½ teaspoon vanilla
½ cup rice flour
¼ cup tapioca flour
¼ cup cornstarch
½ teaspoon salt

FILLING

½ cup sour cream or nondairy substitute
1 3-ounce package cream cheese
¼ cup sugar
1 egg
½ teaspoon vanilla

TOPPING

2 cups peeled, sliced pears
1 tablespoon lemon juice
3 tablespoons brown sugar
1 teaspoon cinnamon
⅓ cup apricot preserves

For the crust, cream together the butter and sugar, then beat in the vanilla. Add the flours, cornstarch, and salt. Blend and press into a greased, deep 9″ pie pan or springform pan. Bake for 10 minutes in a preheated 375° oven. Leave oven on.

Meanwhile, prepare the filling: Beat the sour cream and cream cheese together. Add the sugar, egg, and vanilla, beating until smooth. Pour this over the partially baked crust.

Top with the sliced pears, which have been gently tossed with the lemon juice, brown sugar, and cinnamon. For a more elegant look, arrange the slices in two overlapping circles. Warm the apricot preserves and brush over the pears. Bake at 375° for 45 to 55 minutes, or until golden brown. Cool slightly before serving. (It is also good cold.) *Makes 6 to 8 servings.*

Nutrients per serving: Calories 390, Fat 19 g, Carbohydrate 52 g, Cholesterol 75 mg, Sodium 300 mg, Fiber 2 g, Protein 3 g

Berry Cobbler

350°

This quick-and-easy baked dessert can be made of either fresh or frozen blackberries, loganberries, or blueberries.

1 quart berries
2 cups sugar
2 tablespoons shortening
2 eggs
1 cup GF Mix (page 38)
2 teaspoons baking powder
¼ teaspoon salt
½ cup milk or nondairy liquid
¼ teaspoon vanilla
Whipped cream for garnish

Put berries and 1½ cups sugar in a metal or flameproof 8″ × 10″ baking pan. Over them pour enough water to barely cover the berries. Place the pan on the stove and slowly bring to a boiling point. Meanwhile, mix up the batter.

In a mixing bowl, cream together the remaining ½ cup sugar and the shortening. Beat in the eggs. Sift together the flour, baking powder, and salt; add alternately with the milk. Don't overbeat. Stir in the vanilla.

Drop this by tablespoonfuls over the boiling fruit. Bake in preheated 350° oven for about 25 to 30 minutes. The topping will spread out over the fruit. Serve hot, dishing up topping and fruit together. Garnish with whipped cream. *Makes 8 to 10 servings.*

Nutrients per serving: Calories 300, Fat 6 g, Carbohydrate 61 g, Cholesterol 50 mg, Sodium 160 mg, Fiber 4 g, Protein 3 g

Apple Cheese Crisp

350°

A gluten-free twist to the old crisp that called for oatmeal. Try this on your family. Mine loved it.

FILLING

6 cups peeled, sliced apples (4 to 5 apples)
1¼ teaspoons cinnamon
¼ teaspoon nutmeg
Dash of salt
1 cup sugar
1 tablespoon lemon juice

TOPPING

1 cup GF Mix (page 38)
½ cup brown sugar
6 tablespoons (¾ stick) butter or margarine
1 cup grated Cheddar cheese

Peel and slice the apples into a large mixing bowl. Tumble with the spices, salt, sugar, and lemon juice. Pour out into a 9″ × 13″ baking pan. In a smaller bowl, place the flour and brown sugar. Cut in the butter until the mixture feels like cornmeal. Then mix in the grated cheese. Crumble this topping over the apples. Bake uncovered in a preheated 350° oven for 1 hour. May be served hot or cold. *Makes 10 to 12 servings.*

Nutrients per serving: Calories 260, Fat 9 g, Carbohydrate 44 g, Cholesterol 25 mg, Sodium 360 mg, Fiber 1 g, Protein 3 g

Rhubarb Crumble

350°

Another twist on the old crisp. Rhubarb lovers beware: This is addictive. Top with yogurt or sour cream for an extra-special dessert.

FILLING

1¼ cups sugar
1 tablespoon tapioca flour
½ teaspoon cinnamon
4 cups sliced fresh rhubarb or one 16-ounce package frozen

TOPPING

¾ cup GF Mix (page 38)
½ cup brown sugar
⅛ teaspoon salt
½ cup (1 stick) butter or margarine
½ cup GF bread crumbs or crushed GF cereal

In a small dish, combine sugar, flour, and cinnamon. Mix this with the rhubarb and place in a shallow 9″ × 9″ baking pan. For the topping, combine flour, sugar, and salt. Cut in the butter. Stir in the bread crumbs. Sprinkle this mixture over the rhubarb. Bake 1 hour in preheated 350° oven. Serve warm. *Makes 8 servings.*

Nutrients per serving: Calories 370, Fat 12 g, Carbohydrate 64 g, Cholesterol 30 mg, Sodium 220 mg, Fiber 1 g, Protein 2 g

Lime Sponge Pudding

325°

The lime gives a new taste to the old lemon sponge. It is cake and pudding made together.

3 eggs
1½ cups milk
2 tablespoons butter or margarine
1 cup sugar
½ cup GF Mix (page 38)
⅓ cup lime juice
1 tablespoon grated lime peel

Separate the eggs. Place the yolks in a medium-sized bowl and the whites in another bowl to whip later.

In a medium saucepan, scald the milk. Then beat the egg yolks and slowly whisk or blend in the milk. Melt the butter and add with the sugar, flour, lime juice, and peel.

Beat the egg whites until stiff and fold them into the lime mixture. Spoon into 8 custard cups and arrange the cups in a 9″ × 13″ baking pan. Add hot water to 1 inch around the cups. Bake 22 to 25 minutes in preheated 325° oven. Serve at room temperature or chilled. *Makes 8 servings.*

Nutrients per serving: Calories 200, Fat 4 g, Carbohydrate 36 g, Cholesterol 90 mg, Sodium 60 mg, Fiber 0, Protein 4 g

Blackberry Dumplings

On our family camping trips, my mother, with four children begging for dessert and no oven, created this top-of-the-stove or over-the-campfire treat. It may be made with huckleberries (the original), blueberries, loganberries, or any other juicy fruit you wish.

SAUCE

1 quart fresh or frozen berries
1 cup water (to barely cover fruit)
1½ cups sugar (or to taste)
1 tablespoon lemon juice

DUMPLINGS

2 tablespoons sugar
3 tablespoons shortening
1 egg
⅓ cup buttermilk or sour milk
½ cup rice flour
⅓ cup potato starch flour
2 teaspoons baking powder
½ teaspoon baking soda
½ teaspoon salt

Place the berries, water, sugar, and lemon juice in a 4-quart saucepan on the stove. Bring to a gentle boil while making the dumplings.

In a mixing bowl, cream the sugar and shortening. Beat in the egg. Stir in the buttermilk alternately with the sifted dry ingredients. Do not overbeat. This will be a fairly stiff dough.

Drop dough by 8 small spoonfuls onto the boiling fruit sauce. Cover, turn to simmer, and cook without peeking for 20 minutes.

Serve hot in small bowls with the fruit sauce spooned over the dumpling. Top with cream, whipped cream, or ice cream. *Makes 8 servings.*

Nutrients per serving: Calories 310, Fat 6 g, Carbohydrate 64 g, Cholesterol 25 mg, Sodium 320 mg, Fiber 5 g, Protein 2 g

Fruit Crêpes with Wine Sauce

325°

Wine sauce can be used with many fruits in many ways. Serve the sauce and fruit over sponge cake, waffles, GF ice cream, or yogurt. The fruit can be a mixture of apples, peaches, bananas, or others.

1 recipe Crêpes (page 215)
1½ to 2 cups cut-up fruit
Lemon juice
4 tablespoons (½ stick) butter or margarine
½ cup dark brown sugar
½ teaspoon cinnamon
¼ teaspoon nutmeg
⅓ cup dry white wine

Make the crêpes and prepare the fruit; squeeze lemon juice over the fruit to keep it from discoloring.

Combine butter, brown sugar, spices, and wine in a small saucepan. Bring to a boil, then turn to simmer, stirring constantly for 10 minutes or until slightly thickened into a syrup.

Roll a small amount of fruit in each crêpe, place crêpes seam side down in a lightly buttered 9″ × 9″ baking dish, and top with the syrup. Bake in a preheated 325° oven for about 15 minutes, or microwave for a few minutes. Serve warm. *Makes 4 to 6 servings.*

Nutrients per serving: Calories 250, Fat 12 g, Carbohydrate 31 g, Cholesterol 85 mg, Sodium 220 mg, Fiber 1 g, Protein 3 g

Baked Apples with Nuts and Raisins

375°

A simple winter dessert spiced up for company.

4 large baking apples
2 tablespoons raisins
2 tablespoons chopped walnuts
1 teaspoon cinnamon
1 tablespoon brown sugar
1 tablespoon butter or margarine
½ cup water

Peel skin from the top of the apples to about 1 inch down. Core the apples, trying not to cut all the way through to the bottom. Arrange in an 8″ × 8″ baking dish.

In a small bowl, combine the raisins, walnuts, cinnamon, and brown sugar. Stuff each apple center with equal amounts of the mixture. Dot the tops with butter. Pour the water around the apples and bake in preheated 375° oven for 45 minutes, or until tender but not mushy, basting occasionally with the juicy water.

Serve warm or cool topped with whipped cream or yogurt. *Makes 4 servings.*

Nutrients per serving: Calories 140, Fat 5 g, Carbohydrate 27 g, Cholesterol 10 mg, Sodium 30 mg, Fiber 2 g, Protein 1 g

Baked Bananas

350°

A fine accompaniment to pork, ham, teriyaki chicken, or curry, or serve them as a dessert. These are simple to prepare and can be made earlier in the day to pop into the oven just before dinner is served. Or bake earlier and serve at room temperature.

4 firm eating bananas or special baking bananas such as plantains
1 cup crushed cornflakes
3 tablespoons honey
3 tablespoons lemon juice

Grease an 8″ × 8″ baking dish generously with butter. Peel bananas and cut in half. Roll each section in the crushed cornflakes, pressing slightly so the banana is thoroughly coated. Arrange banana sections in the baking dish. Stir the honey and lemon juice together and drizzle all the sections with the mixture, making sure the bananas are coated.

Bake in preheated 350° oven for 20 minutes. Serve hot or at room temperature. *Makes 4 servings.*

Nutrients per serving: Calories 240, Fat ½ g, Carbohydrate 58 g, Cholesterol 0, Sodium 70 mg, Fiber 6 g, Protein 3 g

Hot Curried Fruit

350°

This spicy mixed-fruit casserole from Jan Winkelman is a fine accompaniment for chicken and rice. Or try it at a brunch to complement ham and sweet rolls.

One 16-ounce can peach halves
One 16-ounce can pear halves
One 13½-ounce can sliced pineapple or pineapple chunks
¼ cup (½ stick) margarine
½ cup brown sugar
1 teaspoon curry powder
Maraschino cherries, for garnish

Drain the fruits, saving the juice. Arrange the fruit attractively in a shallow casserole dish.

In a saucepan, mix together ¼ cup of the reserved fruit juice, the margarine, brown sugar, and curry powder. Heat until the margarine melts. Pour over the fruit and bake in preheated 350° oven for about

30 minutes. Garnish with the cherries before serving hot. *Makes 6 to 8 servings.*

If a larger casserole of fruit is desired, add one 17-ounce can of apricot halves to the above recipe and increase the curry to 1¼ teaspoons powder, or to taste. *Makes 8 to 10 servings.*

Nutrients per serving: Calories 130, Fat 5 g, Carbohydrate 23 g, Cholesterol 10 mg, Sodium 55 mg, Fiber 2 g, Protein 1 g

Wine Curried Fruit

350°

This is a much larger and more elegant casserole of curried fruit to serve at a dinner or buffet.

2 bananas
One 29-ounce can peach halves
One 26-ounce can pear halves
One 20-ounce can pineapple chunks
Two 6½-ounce cans mandarin oranges
One 8-ounce jar maraschino cherries
½ cup (1 stick) butter
½ cup brown sugar
1 tablespoon cornstarch
½ cup dry white wine
1 teaspoon curry powder

Slice the bananas diagonally in 1½-inch chunks. Drain all the other fruit and arrange all in a 2½-quart baking dish. Combine the butter, sugar, cornstarch, wine, and curry powder in a saucepan and cook, stirring constantly, until slightly thickened. Pour over the fruit. Bake, uncovered, in preheated 350° oven for about 15 to 20 minutes. Serve hot. *Makes 12 to 14 servings.*

Nutrients per serving: Calories 190, Fat 7 g, Carbohydrate 34 g, Cholesterol 20 mg, Sodium 75 mg, Fiber 2 g, Protein 1 g

Holiday Fare

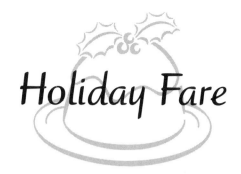

Christmas

Hanukkah

See Also

For most of us holidays have always been associated with food, from that celebratory glass of champagne with hors d'oeuvres to begin the New Year to the final bite of plum pudding on Christmas. If you are like me, the first fear after starting the diet was that the holidays were going to be a food fiasco. Put those worries aside. Pour that champagne (or seltzer water) and toast the New Year with a wide assortment of gluten-free appetizers and go on through the year to greet each holiday in season with your favorite foods.

In this chapter you'll find many of them, for they all convert to gluten free with very little effort and almost no change in taste. There's cherry pie for Presidents' Day and stuffing for the holiday turkey, and in between there's a whole section of recipes for that summer picnic, family gathering, or Fourth of July at the park. You may not be able to sample the casseroles others bring, but you'll have enough choices here that you can bring your own and feast well.

New Year's Eve and Day

The celebrating of a new year is most often a movable feast, with one hand holding a glass and the other picking from a buffet of appetizers. Here's a wide array ranging from a quick-and-easy spread for triangles of GF bread to some filling meat or chicken nibbles that can still be picked up with a toothpick. Finish with a dessert-type party mix.

If you need something more filling for that gang watching the game on New Year's, try the Shrimp Cheese Spread (page 254) atop either split English muffins or slices of bread. It can be mixed up ahead of time, spread as needed, and broiled for a few minutes. You won't miss any of the party!

Savory Chicken Puffs

450°

Fabulous finger food for any buffet. With a zingy taste of chicken, nuts, and seasonings, these are sure to make a hit with your guests. They may be made a day ahead and heated in the microwave before serving.

1½ cups finely chopped cooked chicken
⅓ cup chopped almonds, toasted
⅔ cup rice flour
⅓ cup potato starch
1 cup chicken broth
½ cup shortening
2 teaspoons Worcestershire sauce
1 tablespoon dried parsley
1 teaspoon seasoned salt
¾ teaspoon celery seed
Dash of cayenne pepper
4 eggs

Preheat oven to 450°. Grease two baking sheets.

In a medium bowl, combine the chicken and nuts. Set aside.

In a measuring cup, blend the rice flour and potato starch. Set aside.

In a large saucepan, place the chicken broth, shortening, Worcestershire sauce, parsley, seasoning salt, celery seed, and cayenne pepper. Bring to a boil over high heat. Add the flours all at once and stir until a smooth ball forms. Remove from the heat and let stand 3 minutes.

Add the eggs, one at a time, beating until smooth after each addition. Stir in the chicken and nuts and drop by heaping teaspoonfuls onto the prepared baking sheets. Bake at 450° for 14 minutes, or until golden brown. Serve warm. *Makes 6 dozen puffs.*

Nutrients per puff: Calories 35, Fat 2½ g, Carbohydrate 2 g, Cholesterol 15 mg, Sodium 50 mg, Fiber 0, Protein 1 g

Sausage Cheese Balls 375°

Make this easy baked meat entree for that New Year's buffet table and watch your guests dig in. They'll never guess that you used a GF biscuit mix as the base.

1 pound uncooked sausage (pork or turkey)
¼ cup finely chopped onion
¼ cup finely diced celery
¼ teaspoon garlic powder
8 ounces sharp Cheddar cheese, grated (2 cups)
1 cup Biscuit Mix (page 84)

Preheat oven to 375°.

Place sausage in a large bowl and with your hands work in the onion, celery, and garlic powder. Add the cheese and work that in. Add the biscuit mix. This will take some time to work in evenly and for the meat and cheese to absorb the flour.

Form into 1-inch balls and bake on ungreased cookie sheets until golden brown (15 to 18 minutes). Remove immediately. Store in refrigerator and microwave to reheat before serving if using within 24 hours. Freeze if serving later. Serving size: 3 meatballs. *Makes 3 dozen meatballs.*

Nutrients per serving: Calories 80, Fat 5 g, Carbohydrate 3 g, Cholesterol 15 mg, Sodium 140 mg, Fiber 0, Protein 4 g

Carol's Secret Appetizer 450°

When Carol admitted how simple the ingredients were for her appetizer, those who had tasted them were amazed.

¾ cup mayonnaise
⅓ cup parmesan cheese
⅓ cup finely minced onion (Use food processor or blender)
8 to 10 slices Challah (page 65) or Almost Pumpernickel (page 68)

Preheat oven to 450°.

In a small bowl, combine the mayonnaise, cheese, and onion.

Quarter the bread slices into squares or triangles, spread with the topping, and place on an ungreased cookie sheet. Bake for 3 minutes. Serve hot. *Makes 32 to 40 appetizers.*

Nutrients per appetizer: Calories 50, Fat 2½ g, Carbohydrate 6 g, Cholesterol 5 mg, Sodium 95 mg, Fiber 0, Protein 2 g

White Chocolate Party Mix

Try this as a "finger" dessert. The basic ingredients are not sweet, but they're covered with a sweet white chocolate–like coating. The recipe can be doubled for a large crowd.

Many suppliers have the GF pretzels. You may find other rice square cereals that are GF.

5 ounces GF pretzels
4 cups Health Valley Rice Crunch-Ems
1 cup raisins
1 cup peanuts
8 ounces M&Ms
One 12-ounce package vanilla chips
1½ tablespoons vegetable oil

In a large bowl, combine the pretzels, Crunch-Ems, raisins, peanuts, and M&Ms.

In a medium saucepan (or in a microwavable bowl in the microwave), melt the chips and oil until smooth. Pour over the mix and stir until well coated. Spoon onto wax paper and cool. Store in an airtight container. *Makes 2½ quarts, 16 to 20 servings.*

Nutrients per serving: Calories 280, Fat 14 g, Carbohydrate 35 g, Cholesterol 5 mg, Sodium 190 mg, Fiber 1 g, Protein 4 g

Presidents' Day

Cherry Cheese Pie

It's hard to believe something so good could be so easy. A fine dessert for the holiday.

One 8-ounce package cream cheese
One 14-ounce can sweetened condensed milk
⅓ cup lemon juice
1 teaspoon vanilla
1 Cereal Crust (page 148) or Crumb Crust (page 148)
One 21-ounce can GF cherry pie filling

In a mixing bowl, soften the cream cheese, then beat until fluffy. Beat in the sweetened condensed milk until smooth. Stir in the lemon juice and vanilla. Pour into the prepared crust. Chill 3 hours or until set. Top with pie filling. Keep pie refrigerated. *Makes 6 to 8 servings.*

Nutrients per serving: Calories 430, Fat 19 g, Carbohydrate 60 g, Cholesterol 60 mg, Sodium 270 mg, Fiber 0, Protein 7 g

Easter

Hot Cross Buns

380°

You don't have to miss this Easter favorite now that you're on the gluten-free diet. These will taste like the ones you remember.

2 cups Four Flour Bean Mix (pages 38–39)
1½ teaspoons xanthan gum
1 teaspoon unflavored gelatin
½ teaspoon salt
3 tablespoons brown sugar
¾ teaspoon cinnamon or cardamom
1 teaspoon Egg Replacer
2 tablespoons dry milk powder or nondairy substitute
2 eggs
2 tablespoons margarine or butter
¾ teaspoon dough enhancer or vinegar
2¼ teaspoons dry yeast granules
¾ cup warm water (110°–115°)
½ teaspoon granulated sugar
⅓ cup raisins, dried cranberries, or citron (or a combination)

Grease an 8″ square pan and dust with rice flour.

In a medium bowl, combine the flour mix, xanthan gum, gelatin, salt, brown sugar, cinnamon, Egg Replacer, and dry milk powder. Set aside.

In the bowl of a heavy-duty mixer, place the eggs, margarine (cut into small chunks), and dough enhancer. Beat at medium speed until the eggs are frothy.

Dissolve the yeast in the water to which the granulated sugar has been added. When frothy, add to the egg mixture. With the mixer on low, spoon in the dry ingredients. Beat on high for 2 minutes. Stir in the fruit and spoon into the prepared pan in 3 rows of 3 round, bun-shaped spoonfuls. Cover and let rise about 35 minutes for rapid-rising yeast or about 60 minutes for regular yeast, or until almost double in bulk. *Makes 9 buns.*

Bake in a preheated 380° oven for approximately 28 minutes. For a finishing touch, combine ¾ cup confectioners' sugar with 1 to 2 tablespoons orange juice or milk and pipe this icing in the form of a cross on each bun when cooled.

Nutrients per bun: Calories 190, Fat 4 g, Carbohydrate 34 g, Cholesterol 30 mg, Sodium 180 mg, Fiber 2 g, Protein 5 g

Cinco de Mayo

Even in my Pacific Rim part of the country, the Fifth of May is celebrated with food and parties.

Burrito Wraps

We may not be able to buy a burrito at the nearest Mexican take-out, but you can throw your own burrito party gluten free. These wraps are as easy to make as a pancake and taste great when rolled around any kind of filling.

1 cup Four Flour Bean Mix (pages 38–39)
½ teaspoon salt
¼ teaspoon xanthan gum
½ cup liquid egg substitute
1½ cups water
1 tablespoon margarine or butter, melted

In a medium bowl, whisk together the flour mix, salt, and xanthan gum. Add the egg substitute and about ¼ cup of the water. Beat together until smooth. Slowly beat in the rest of the water. Stir in the melted margarine. Place bowl in the refrigerator and let rest for at least 20 minutes.

Heat a 9″ skillet or frypan over high heat and brush lightly with oil. Be sure it is hot enough for water to dance on the surface before starting to cook the wraps. Using a ⅓ cup measure, pour in the batter and quickly tilt the pan to cover all the bottom surface. Cook until the bottom of the wrap is dry and the top is almost dry. Turn and barely cook the other side. Slip onto wax paper. Repeat the process.

Store, separated by wax paper, in a plastic bag in the refrigerator or freezer until ready to use. *Makes eight 8-inch wraps.*

Nutrients per serving: Calories 110, Fat 2 g, Carbohydrate 20 g, Cholesterol 5 mg, Sodium 160 mg, Fiber 1 g, Protein 1 g

Rice Flour Tortillas

Finally! A flour tortilla for those who can't have wheat. These are made in the traditional way by flattening and rolling, then cooking on a hot griddle. Use them for enchiladas, burritos, or fajitas. These keep well in the refrigerator or freezer.

2 cups GF Mix (page 38)
1½ teaspoons xanthan gum
2 teaspoons sugar
1 teaspoon salt
2 teaspoons milk powder or nondairy substitute
1 cup warm water

In the bowl of a mixer, blend flour mix, xanthan gum, sugar, salt, and milk powder. Add the water and beat on medium speed for 1 minute.

Remove dough from mixer and form a ball. Divide into 6 or 8 parts and, working on cornstarch-dusted plastic wrap, roll out each piece very thin until it forms a 10″ to 12″ round. Roll all the pieces, separating them with plastic wrap or wax paper before cooking.

Heat a griddle to medium-hot or hot and cook each tortilla about 1 minute per side. *Makes 6 large or 8 medium tortillas.*

Nutrients per serving: Calories 190, Fat ½ g, Carbohydrate 44 g, Cholesterol 0 g, Sodium 5 mg, Fiber 1 g, Protein 2 g

Fillings for Burritos

To throw a burrito party, all it takes is a stack of GF tortillas plus bowls of the following:

Shredded lettuce
Grated cheese
Chopped tomatoes
Refried beans or mashed, cooked pinto beans seasoned with enchilada sauce
Salsa
Green onions, chopped
Yogurt, sour cream, guacamole
Enchilada sauce (optional)

NOTE: Some grocery stores now carry shredded pork and chicken in a sauce and many are gluten-free. Add them to the list for your party.

Let the guests pick their fillings, roll the burritos, and eat with their hands.

Fourth of July and Summer Picnics

Whether it's the annual picnic in the park or a family gathering, you're not going to be able to eat many of those offerings that others bring. So make and take casseroles and dishes you can eat and watch the others enjoy them, too.

Barbecued Spareribs

What's a summer picnic without the barbecue going? Usually we have to pass up any item like this because of the sauce, but if we make our own, we can eat safely. These may also be broiled and roasted if the weather is not fit for barbecuing.

4 pounds pork spareribs
Water
½ cup sliced onion
1¼ cups ketchup
3 tablespoons fruit vinegar (cranberry, raspberry, or apple)
2 tablespoons dark corn syrup
2 teaspoons salt
1 teaspoon paprika
¾ teaspoon chili powder

Precook the spareribs, drain, and chill before barbecuing, broiling, or baking.

Cut the spareribs into 2 or 3 rib portions and place in a large kettle. Add cold water to cover and the sliced onion. Bring to a boil over high heat, reduce to low, cover, and simmer for 1 hour. Drain, cover, and chill until ready to grill.

Sauce: In a medium bowl, combine the ketchup, vinegar, corn syrup, salt, paprika, and chili powder.

Barbecuing: Place ribs on grill over medium coals. Brush often with sauce and turn occasionally. Grill 20 minutes.

Broiling and roasting: Place ribs on broiler pan. Brush with sauce and broil about 5 minutes on each side. Turn oven to 400° and finish baking, about 10 to 15 minutes. Brush about every 5 minutes with sauce. *Serves 4.*

Nutrients per serving: Calories 970, Fat 69 g, Carbohydrate 18 g, Cholesterol 275 mg, Sodium 1300 mg, Fiber 1 g, Protein 67 g

Potato Salad

Even when I couldn't cook, my potato salads won praise. I now realize potato salad is one dish that is gluten free naturally as long as GF mayonnaise is used. It can be eaten without aftereffects. Most of the ones in the deli are not gluten free, so I still go on making my own version.

NOTE: I choose potatoes that are firm and do not cook down. Some of the best are Yukon Gold and red potatoes. Do not use a baking potato.

5 fist-sized potatoes
5 eggs
4 to 6 tablespoons sweet pickle relish (or to taste)
1 medium onion, finely diced
Salt and pepper to taste
¾ cup mayonnaise
⅓ cup evaporated milk or nondairy substitute
2 teaspoons prepared mustard
Paprika (optional)

Boil the potatoes and eggs together in salted water. Twenty minutes is usually enough time, but test to be sure the potatoes are done. Drain and set aside to cool completely.

Dice the potatoes and 4 of the eggs. Layer the salad with the potatoes, eggs, pickle relish, onion, salt, and pepper. (This is to prevent too much tumbling and stirring that breaks up the potatoes.) Stir gently.

Make the dressing: Thin the mayonnaise with the milk and add the mustard. Blend well. Stir gently into the salad. Top with the last egg, sliced, and sprinkle with paprika if desired. Cover well and refrigerate for at least 8 hours or overnight for the flavors to meld. *Makes 8 to 10 servings.*

Nutrients per serving: Calories 270, Fat 18 g, Carbohydrate 24 g, Cholesterol 115 mg, Sodium 270 mg, Fiber 1 g, Protein 6 g

Baked Beans with a Nip 375°

This easy-to-make bean dish is another winner at gatherings and potlucks. It uses some different canned beans and has the added nip of chili for a twist.

5 ounces bacon, cut in ½-inch pieces
2 cups chopped onions
One 16-ounce can tomato sauce
1 cup brown sugar
6 tablespoons apple cider vinegar
3 tablespoons molasses
1 tablespoon Worcestershire sauce
2 teaspoons chili powder (or to taste)
5 drops hot pepper sauce
One (16-ounce) can garbanzo beans, drained
One (16-ounce) can kidney beans, drained
One (16-ounce) can black beans, drained
One (16-ounce) can butter beans, drained

Preheat oven to 375°.

In a large ovenproof pot, sauté the bacon and onions until the bacon is brown and the onions translucent. Mix in tomato sauce, sugar, vinegar, molasses, Worcestershire sauce, chili powder, and hot pepper sauce. Rinse the beans thoroughly and add. Cover the pot and bake for about 1 hour and 30 minutes, stirring occasionally. *Makes 8 to 10 servings.*

Nutrients per serving: Calories 340, Fat 4 g, Carbohydrate 66 g, Cholesterol 5 mg, Sodium 820 mg, Fiber 9 g, Protein 13 g

Garlic Dills

If you're hesitant about eating pickles made with an unknown source of vinegar, why not make your own. These are so easy—and delicious!

6 pounds 3- to 5-inch pickling cucumbers
Ice water to soak
3 cups apple cider vinegar
6 cups water
½ cup pickling salt
12 to 24 heads fresh dill
12 cloves garlic

Wash cucumbers and remove 1⁄16 inch from the blossom end. Soak in ice water for 24 hours, checking the ice every 8 hours or so. Drain.

Wash 12 pint jars or 6 quart jars and scald. Place 1 to 2 heads of dill and 1 to 2 cloves of garlic in each hot jar. Firmly pack the cucumbers into the jars, leaving ½ inch headspace. (If the cucumbers are too fat, cut lengthwise into quarters for closer packing.) Top with an additional 1 to 2 heads of dill.

In a large (4- to 6-quart) saucepan, combine the vinegar, water, and pickling salt. Bring to a boil over high heat and immediately pour into the jars over the cucumbers, leaving ½ inch headspace. Wipe the jar tops and threads clean and top with the lids. Screw down the bands firmly.

Process in boiling water canner for 15 minutes. For pickles to develop full flavor, let stand 2 to 3 weeks before opening and eating. *Makes 6 quarts or 12 pints.*

Nutrients per ½ pickle: Calories 0, Fat 0, Carbohydrate 0, Cholesterol 0, Sodium 210 mg, Fiber 1 g, Protein 0

Halloween

How times have changed! Now it isn't only the children who dress in costumes and party on this night.

Oven Caramel Corn

200°

A great snack for that fall or Halloween party!

20 cups popcorn
2 cups brown sugar
1 cup butter or margarine
½ cup light corn syrup
½ teaspoon salt
½ teaspoon baking soda
2 cups pecan halves

Preheat oven to 200°. Grease a large roaster and pour in the popcorn.

In a medium saucepan, combine the brown sugar, butter, corn syrup, and salt. Cook over medium heat, stirring occasionally, until mixture reaches a full boil. Continue cooking until the soft ball stage, or 238° on a candy thermometer. Remove from the heat and stir in the baking soda. Pour over the popcorn. Sprinkle on the pecans and stir until well mixed. Bake for 20 minutes. Stir again and bake another 25 minutes. Remove from oven and stir again before spreading out on cookie sheets. When cool, break into bite-sized pieces. *Makes 30 to 40 servings.*

Nutrients per serving: Calories 150, Fat 9 g, Carbohydrate 18 g, Cholesterol 15 mg, Sodium 170 mg, Fiber 1 g, Protein 1 g

Thanksgiving

Thanksgiving is one of the few holidays that hasn't been changed in our commercial economy. It's still a time of family, friends, and familiar food.

Old-fashioned Pumpkin Pie 425°/350°

We've put pumpkin in breads and mousses, and fluffed it into chiffon pies, but most true pumpkin pie lovers still ask for old-fashioned pie for their Thanksgiving dessert.

2 eggs
One 16-ounce can pumpkin
¾ cup sugar
½ teaspoon salt
2 teaspoons pumpkin pie spice
1½ cups cream or nondairy substitute
1 Cereal Crust (page 148)

In a large mixing bowl, beat the eggs slightly. Add pumpkin, sugar, salt, and spice. Stir together. Add the cream and mix thoroughly. Pour into the unbaked crust. Bake in preheated 425° oven for 15 minutes. Reduce temperature to 350° and bake another 45 minutes, or until a knife inserted in the center of the pie comes out clean. Cool.

Serve cold with whipped cream or whipped nondairy topping if desired. *Makes 6 to 8 servings.*

Nutrients per serving: Calories 300, Fat 12 g, Carbohydrate 44 g, Cholesterol 90 mg, Sodium 400 mg, Fiber 0, Protein 4 g

Orange Cornbread Stuffing

Roast turkey with sausage and orange cornbread dressing was a traditional Thanksgiving favorite in the Old South. It's excellent, too, for those on a gluten-free diet. But don't save it just for Thanksgiving. Use it with Cornish game hens, roast chicken, or pork (eliminating the sausage).

1 recipe Orange Cornbread (page 88)
½ pound bulk pork sausage (optional)
1 medium onion, diced
½ cup chopped green pepper (optional)
½ cup sliced celery
2 eggs, beaten
1 teaspoon dried thyme
½ teaspoon salt
1 to 1½ cups chicken stock

Prepare orange cornbread, using only 2 eggs. Cool, crumble, and set aside.

In a large skillet, sauté the sausage if using, onion, green pepper if using, and celery until meat is browned and vegetables just tender. Drain thoroughly.

In a large bowl, combine the sausage mixture, eggs, thyme, and salt. Add the crumbled cornbread and toss until well mixed. Add enough stock to moisten to desired consistency. The full amount of stock will make a moist dressing. If you prefer it drier, cut the amount of liquid.

Makes enough to stuff a 12- to 14-pound bird. Or you may bake it in a greased 2½-quart casserole in preheated 325° oven for about 45 minutes.

Nutrients per serving: Calories 250, Fat 13 g, Carbohydrate 28 g, Cholesterol 110 mg, Sodium 611 mg, Fiber 2 g, Protein 8 g

Rice Bread Stuffing

If you don't want to make the cornbread recipe, you can use up your stale rice bread or use those crumbs salvaged from bread recipes that failed and still have a stuffing everyone will praise.

1 large onion, minced
1 cup diced celery
6 tablespoons (¾ stick) butter or margarine
1 to 1½ teaspoons poultry seasoning
2 tablespoons minced parsley
6 to 8 cups GF bread, crumbled
1 to 1½ cups chicken broth
Salt to taste

Sauté the onion and celery in butter until clear; add the poultry seasoning and parsley. Pour this mixture over the bread in a large mixing bowl. Stir until blended, then add the broth, a little at a time, until the dressing is as moist as you prefer. Add salt to taste. *Makes enough to stuff a 10- to 12-pound turkey.*

SEASONED BREAD: If you are baking your GF bread near the holiday season, try putting the 1 to 1½ teaspoons poultry seasoning directly into the dough for at least one loaf before you bake it. Try adding some dried minced parsley also. This seasoned bread will make excellent stuffing and win you raves. It works best with the True Yeast Bread recipe (page 53), using white rice flour.

Nutrients per serving: Calories 540, Fat 10 g, Carbohydrate 102 g, Cholesterol 20 mg, Sodium 760 mg, Fiber 6 g, Protein 11 g

Pumpkin Roll

375°

Pumpkin pie taste in an easy-to-make cake roll. Make this for a welcome change for your next holiday dinner. This can be made a day (or even two) ahead to save time for your guests on the big day.

¾ cup Four Flour Bean Mix or GF Mix (pages 38–39)
½ teaspoon (scant) xanthan gum
1 teaspoon baking powder
1 teaspoon Egg Replacer (if using GF Mix)
2 teaspoons cinnamon
1 teaspoon ginger
½ teaspoon nutmeg
3 eggs
1 cup sugar
⅔ cup canned pumpkin
1 teaspoon lemon juice
Nondairy whipped topping for filling
1 teaspoon vanilla powder

Preheat oven to 375°. Cut wax paper to fit an 11″ × 16″ jelly roll pan. Grease the pan well; fit paper into pan and grease paper.

In a medium bowl, whisk together the flour, xanthan gum, baking powder, Egg Replacer (if used), cinnamon, ginger, and nutmeg. Set aside.

In a large mixing bowl, beat the eggs and sugar until light. Mix in the pumpkin and lemon juice. Add the dry ingredients and mix well. Pour into the prepared pan, spreading well so the batter is even. Bake at 375° for 15 minutes.

Cool 15 minutes before turning out onto a clean, flat-textured tea towel that has been rubbed with powdered sugar. Remove the paper and roll up (from the 11-inch side) in the towel, folding some of the towel over the cake at the beginning. Let cool. Unroll and fill with a thick spread of nondairy whipped topping flavored with the powdered vanilla. Reroll without the towel and seal in foil. Refrigerate until serving. *Makes 8 servings.*

Nutrients per serving: Calories 180, Fat 2½ g, Carbohydrate 38 g, Cholesterol 80 mg, Sodium 75 mg, Fiber 1 g, Protein 4 g

Christmas

For many, the foods of the Christmas season are handed down in the family just as the beloved old ornaments for the tree are treasured.

Christmas Stollen

375°

An excellent Christmas bread. This uses no yeast, but the ricotta cheese assures lightness and great taste.

3 cups Four Flour Bean Mix or GF Mix (pages 38–39)
2½ teaspoons xanthan gum
4 teaspoons baking powder
1 teaspoon baking soda
¼ teaspoon salt
⅔ cup sugar
2 cups ricotta cheese
2 tablespoons margarine or butter, melted
4 eggs, slightly beaten
¼ to ⅓ cup buttermilk
3 tablespoons candied fruit mix
2 tablespoons golden raisins
2 tablespoons chopped almonds
1 tablespoon grated lemon peel

Preheat oven to 375°. Grease a large cookie sheet and dust with rice flour.

In the bowl of your mixer combine flour mix, xanthan gum, baking powder, baking soda, salt, and sugar. Blend on low. Add the ricotta cheese, melted margarine, and beaten eggs. Beat until well blended. The dough will be very thick. Add enough of the buttermilk to make it the texture of soft cookie dough. Beat for 2½ minutes. Stir in the candied fruit mix, raisins, almonds, and lemon peel. Spoon out onto the cookie sheet in one 12-inch loaf. Bake at 375° for 50 to 60 minutes, covering with aluminum foil after the first 20 minutes. Remove from baking sheet and, if desired, rub the loaf with margarine or butter for a shiny look and tender crust. Cool completely before slicing. *Makes 20 slices.*

Nutrients per slice: Calories 160, Fat 5 g, Carbohydrate 24 g, Cholesterol 50 mg, Sodium 180 mg, Fiber 1 g, Protein 4 g

Cranberry Cheesecake with Pecan Crust 350°

Try this as a colorful and different dessert on that holiday table. It's been lightened considerably compared to most cheesecakes, and the tangy topping is perfect to end the meal. Better yet, this can be made two days ahead to free your time on the holiday.

CRUST

1 cup GF cookie or bread crumbs
⅓ cup ground pecans
1 tablespoon sugar (2 to 3 if using bread crumbs)
3 tablespoons margarine or butter, melted

FILLING

8 ounces one-third fat reduced cream cheese
2 cups fat-free cottage cheese
1 cup fat-free sour cream
1½ cups sugar
3 eggs
1 tablespoon grated orange zest
1 teaspoon orange or vanilla flavoring
¼ cup GF Mix (page 38)

TOPPING

3 tablespoons orange juice
½ cup sugar
1½ cups fresh or frozen cranberries
1 tablespoon cornstarch
2 tablespoons water

Preheat oven to 350°. Grease a 9″ springform pan with vegetable oil spray.

Crust: In a plastic bag, blend the crumbs, ground nuts, sugar, and margarine. Pat into the prepared pan and bake for 8 minutes. Cool and wrap the bottom and sides well with aluminum foil.

Filling: In a food processor, process the cream cheese and cottage cheese until smooth. Add the sour cream, sugar, eggs, orange zest, flavoring, and flour mix. Process until well blended and light. Pour over the baked crust. Place pan in a larger pan and fill this with boiling water until halfway up the sides of springform pan.

Bake 1 hour and 10 minutes. Turn oven off and leave cake in oven for 30 minutes more with the door shut. Remove from water and cool. Refrigerate.

Topping: In a medium saucepan, blend the orange juice and sugar. Bring to a boil for 2 minutes. Add berries, return to a boil, lower heat, and simmer 1 minute. In a small bowl, blend the cornstarch and water. Stir into the berries. Boil, stirring, until thickened. Cool and then spread over cooled cake. Refrigerate until serving. *Makes 12 to 16 servings.*

Nutrients per serving: Calories 230, Fat 7 g, Carbohydrate 33 g, Cholesterol 55 mg, Sodium 230 mg, Fiber 1 g, Protein 8 g

Tropical Fruitcake 250°

This rich, moist fruitcake is pure fruit and nuts.

2¼ cups pecans
1¾ cups walnuts
1 pound pitted dates
8 ounces candied cherries
8 ounces candied pineapple
4 ounces shredded coconut or macadamia nuts
One 14-ounce can sweetened condensed milk

Preheat oven to 250°. Grease three 3″ × 6″ loaf pans and dust with rice flour.

Chop the pecans, walnuts, and dates. Cut up the cherries and pineapple. Slice the macadamia nuts (if used).

Combine pecans, walnuts, dates, cherries, pineapple, coconut or macadamia nuts, and condensed milk. Mix with hands.

Pack tightly into prepared loaf pans. Bake in preheated 250° oven for about 3 hours. Cake is done when no milk oozes out when pressed with fingers.

Cool in pans turned on their side. Remove and wrap snugly in foil. Store in refrigerator or freezer about 1 month before serving. *Makes 30 slices.*

Nutrients per serving: Calories 180, Fat 9 g, Carbohydrate 25 g, Cholesterol 5 mg, Sodium 25 mg, Fiber 2 g, Protein 3 g

Christmas Fruitcake 300°

This excellent fruitcake is more spicy and cakelike than the preceding one. It also stores and freezes well. The taste will vary according to the mincemeat used and the types of fruit and nuts.

2 eggs
28 ounces (2⅔ cups) mincemeat (see Note)
One 14-ounce can sweetened condensed milk
1 pound candied fruits
1 cup chopped walnuts or pecans
2 cups rice flour
½ cup soy flour
½ teaspoon xanthan gum
1 teaspoon salt
2½ teaspoons baking powder
1 teaspoon baking soda

Preheat oven to 300°. Grease two 8½″ × 4½″ loaf pans or a 12-cup ring baking pan and dust with rice flour.

In a large mixing bowl, beat the eggs slightly. Add the mincemeat, condensed milk, candied fruits, and nuts. Mix together the flours, xanthan gum, salt, baking powder, and baking soda. Fold the dry mixture into the fruit mixture.

Pour into prepared pan(s). Bake for 2 hours. Cool in pan. Remove and store in refrigerator or freezer. *Makes 30 slices.*

Nutrients per serving: Calories 300, Fat 26 g, Carbohydrate 64 g, Cholesterol 31 mg, Sodium 115 mg, Fiber 1 g, Protein 2 g

NOTE: Check ingredient list. Some mincemeats contain wheat starch flour, others cornstarch. I have used the dried mincemeat that you reconstitute with water and find it works well.

Mock Mince Pie

400°

A light substitute for old-fashioned mincemeat pie. My tasters all agreed it was excellent.

1 recipe Vinegar Pastry (Revised), page 146
1⅓ cups sugar
½ teaspoon salt
½ teaspoon cinnamon
¼ teaspoon cloves
¼ teaspoon ginger
2 cups peeled, chopped apple
1 cup raisins
One 8-ounce can cranberry sauce
⅓ cup chopped walnuts or pecans
1 teaspoon dried orange peel
1 teaspoon dried lemon peel
3 tablespoons lemon juice
1 tablespoon milk for brushing
½ teaspoon sugar for brushing

Preheat oven to 400°.

Prepare pastry and fit bottom crust into a deep 9″ pie pan.

Place all remaining ingredients in a large mixing bowl and toss together lightly. Place in the piecrust. Top with the second crust. Cut vents. Brush the top with 1 tablespoon milk and ½ teaspoon sugar and bake for 30 to 35 minutes. Serve warm. *Makes 6 servings.*

Nutrients per serving: Calories 840, Fat 31 g, Carbohydrate 140 g, Cholesterol 35 mg, Sodium 520 mg, Fiber 4 g, Protein 5 g

Mother's Plum Pudding

Plum pudding was a Christmas tradition in our house. This recipe, handed down from my mother's English family, made an instant hit with everyone when I converted it to rice and soy flours. My guests now ask for this rather than the original recipe. It is inexpensive, light, and moist. Like all plum puddings, it can be made several days ahead, thus saving the cook's time for enjoying Christmas.

¾ cup rice flour
¾ cup soy flour
1 rounded teaspoon baking soda
½ teaspoon salt
1 teaspoon each cinnamon, nutmeg, and cloves
1½ cups brown sugar
1 cup raisins
1½ cups chopped raw cranberries (see Notes)
1 cup ground suet
1 cup ground raw carrots
1 cup ground raw potatoes

Sift together flours, baking soda, salt, and spices. Blend in brown sugar. Stir in fruit, suet, carrots, and potatoes.

Grease a 2-quart mold (see Notes). Fill three-quarters full and cap with the top. Put mold in a deep dutch oven or soup pot in enough water to maintain steam around it for 3 hours of cooking on top of the stove. This should be covered, and no peeking except to check water. Be sure it doesn't boil away. You should be able to maintain steam by setting the stove at simmer or low.

Store pudding in refrigerator after cooling. It keeps well for a week or more or can be frozen if made earlier. Serve, reheated, with whipped cream or hard sauce. *Serves 16 to 20.*

NOTES: The original recipe used tart apples, but when cranberries became a popular holiday item, my mother switched to them. You may use apples if you prefer.

Three 19-ounce cans can replace the pudding mold. Seal tops with wax paper and aluminum foil and secure with rubber bands.

Nutrients per serving: Calories 180, Fat 11 g, Carbohydrate 46 g, Cholesterol 10 mg, Sodium 180 mg, Fiber 2 g, Protein 2 g

Hanukkah

Latkes (Potato Pancakes)

Potato pancakes have always been a Hanukkah tradition. Little girls learned how to grate the potatoes and test the texture at their mother's side in the Jewish kitchen. It was hard work, but with the food processor, most of the work is taken out of this dish. It's too good to save just for the holiday.

3 fist-sized potatoes
1 onion about 2½ inches round
2 eggs
2 tablespoons rice flour
½ teaspoon salt
¼ teaspoon pepper

Peel and quarter the potatoes and place in a bowl of water until ready to process. In the blender, pulse the onion until finely chopped. Remove to a mixing bowl and then pulse the potatoes in several batches until finely chopped. Beat the eggs. Add them with the flour and seasonings to the potatoes and onions. Mix well.

Fry the pancakes in about ¼ inch of hot oil (see Note) until golden, about 3 to 4 minutes per side. Serve hot. *Makes 9 to 10 pancakes.*

NOTE: Traditionally latkes are fried in hot oil, but if you don't mind defying tradition, they turn out delicious cooked on a very lightly greased Teflon pan.

Nutrients per serving: Calories 50, Fat 1 g, Carbohydrate 8 g, Cholesterol 45 mg, Sodium 120 mg, Fiber 1 g, Protein 2 g

Breakfast and Brunch

When I first started cooking gluten free, pancakes seemed to be the only baking that turned out successfully, for I was using rice flour without blending it with other flours. Now, with the blends, there is no reason a gluten-free diet should be restricted to only pancakes at breakfast or brunch. Crêpes, waffles, and coffee cakes can be so good that the rest of the family will enjoy them, too.

In the following section you'll find a wide variety of breakfast and brunch favorites, ranging from a gluten-free muesli to Toad-in-the-Hole.

I use the GF Mix in many of the recipes, and in others I use the Four Flour Bean Mix. Some of the old recipes can be converted to the new mix.

Muesli

There are several gluten-free cereals on the market, but none combine fruit, grain, and protein as does this mixture, which will give variety to the breakfast menu.

3 cups gluten-free puffed rice
1 cup Perky's Nutty Rice cereal or Jowar Jo-Crisps
3 cups gluten-free cornflakes
1 cup roasted soy nuts, peanuts, coconut, or almonds
1 cup sunflower seeds
1 cup each of any 2:
currants or raisins
dried date bits
dried banana flakes
dried cherries or apples
dried peach or apricot bits

Simply toss all ingredients together and store in plastic freezer bags. (No need to freeze, but the freezer bags are thicker.) Great for a hasty breakfast at home or to take on trips so you can have a gluten-free breakfast cereal when there is none on the menu. *Makes 10 cups muesli. Serving size ½ cup.*

Nutrients per serving: Calories 200, Fat 4 g, Carbohydrate 23 g, Cholesterol 0, Sodium 31 mg, Fiber 2 g, Protein 6 g

English Muffins 350°

These yeasty breakfast crumpets are easy to make since you bake them with only 1 rising. They turn out heavy, flat circles of bread that look, smell, and taste like those containing wheat. These freeze well and are an excellent bread for traveling. They also make a fine base for the Shrimp Cheese Spread found *on page 254.*

You will need 12 English muffin rings. If you wish to try the recipe before investing in baking tins, roll out the dough and cut in circles with a 4-inch glass or can and bake the circles on a greased baking sheet.

2 cups rice flour
2 cups tapioca flour
⅔ cup dried milk or nondairy substitute
3½ teaspoons xanthan gum
1 teaspoon salt
2 tablespoons dry yeast granules
1 cup lukewarm water
1 tablespoon sugar
3 tablespoons shortening
½ cup hot water
4 egg whites, at room temperature

Put flours, dried milk, xanthan gum, and salt in mixer bowl. Crumble the yeast into the lukewarm water with the sugar added. Melt the shortening in the hot water.

In mixing bowl, blend the dry ingredients on low. Pour in the hot water and shortening, blending to mix. Add the egg whites, blend again, then add the yeast mixture. Beat on high speed for 4 minutes.

Spoon half the dough onto a rice-floured board or rice-floured wax paper. Sprinkle some rice flour over the top and then roll out to ½ inch thickness. Cut circles with the English muffin tins or your substitute. With a spatula, lift the dough and tins together and place on greased baking sheets. Repeat with the second half of the dough. Let rise, covered, for 35 to 40 minutes for rapid-rising yeast, 60 minutes for regular.

Put the sheets into a preheated 350° oven. Bake for 20 minutes, then, with a spatula, turn the muffins (tins and all) over. Bake another 20 minutes (40 minutes altogether).

Remove from cookie sheets to rack to cool. (You may remove the rings while they are hot.) *Makes twelve 4-inch muffins.*

Nutrients per muffin: Calories 240, Fat 5 g, Carbohydrate 42 g, Cholesterol 80 mg, Sodium 250 mg, Fiber 1 g, Protein 6 g

Buttermilk Pancakes

When a gourmet friend said she never made pancakes unless she had buttermilk on hand, I thought of trying to create a recipe with our gluten-free flour. She declared these a success. (I didn't tell her that I used powdered buttermilk.) You can use all rice flour instead of the GF Mix if you prefer.

1 cup GF Mix (page 38)
¼ cup buttermilk powder
1 tablespoon sugar
1 teaspoon baking powder
½ teaspoon baking soda
½ teaspoon salt
2 eggs
1 cup water
2 tablespoons vegetable oil

Whisk the dry ingredients together in a mixing bowl. Beat the eggs with the water and oil and add to the dry ingredients. Beat until the batter is smooth, but do not overbeat.

Drop from a mixing spoon onto a hot greased griddle and cook until the top is full of tiny bubbles and the underside is brown. Turn and brown on the other side. *Makes ten 4-inch pancakes.* (Recipe can easily be doubled.)

Nutrients per pancake: Calories 280, Fat 10 g, Carbohydrate 39 g, Cholesterol 110 mg, Sodium 140 mg, Fiber 1 g, Protein 7 g

Rice-Ricotta Pancakes ✓

A crêpelike pancake with delicate texture and flavor—delicious. This batter can be made either in a food processor or with an electric mixer. For a thicker pancake, reduce the milk to ½ cup.

2 eggs
½ cup ricotta cheese
1 tablespoon vegetable oil
½ cup rice flour
2 teaspoons sugar

1 teaspoon baking powder
½ teaspoon salt
¾ cup milk or nondairy
 liquid

Beat together the eggs and ricotta cheese and add the oil. In a large measuring cup, mix flour, sugar, baking powder, and salt. Beat into egg mixture alternately with the milk. The mixture will be thin. Pour onto either lightly greased or Teflon griddle and bake at medium high. (Too hot a griddle will burn the pancakes.) *Makes 1 dozen 4-inch pancakes.*

Nutrients per pancake: Calories 110, Fat 6 g, Carbohydrate 11 g, Cholesterol 65 mg, Sodium 230 mg, Fiber 0, Protein 5 g

Buttermilk Waffles

An easy-to-make waffle for the whole family. No one will guess it is gluten free. The baked waffles freeze well, to be used later under creamed meat sauces or as a shortcake for fruit. You may use Four-Flour Bean Mix in place of the GF Mix.

1¼ cups GF Mix
 (page 38) (see Notes)
¼ cup buttermilk powder
2 teaspoons baking powder
1 teaspoon baking soda

½ teaspoon salt
1 tablespoon sugar
3 tablespoons shortening
2 eggs
1 cup water

✓

Sift the dry ingredients into a mixing bowl. Cut in the shortening until the mixture is very fine. In another bowl, beat the eggs and water. Add these to the dry ingredients. Beat just until the batter is smooth; do not overbeat. Bake on a hot waffle iron. *Makes 3 or 4 waffles.*

NOTES: All white rice flour may be used, or a combination of ¾ cup rice flour and ½ cup corn flour. Each makes a slightly different-tasting waffle.

For a lighter waffle, separate the eggs.

Beat the yolks with the water. Beat the whites to soft peaks and fold into the batter after the final beating.

Nutrients per waffle: Calories 270, Fat 13 g, Carbohydrate 35 g, Cholesterol 105 mg, Sodium 800 mg, Fiber 1 g, Protein 8 g

Rice-Soy Waffles

A light, crisp waffle, easy to make. For a lighter waffle, separate the eggs. Beat the whites to soft peaks and fold into the batter after the dry ingredients.

1 cup rice flour
½ cup soy flour
½ cup potato starch flour
½ teaspoon salt
5 teaspoons baking powder
1 tablespoon sugar
3 eggs
¼ cup vegetable oil
1½ cups milk or nondairy liquid

Measure dry ingredients, mix together, and set aside.

In a mixing bowl, beat eggs, oil, and milk. Add dry ingredients and fold in gently with spoon. Don't overbeat.

Bake on a heated waffle iron and serve. These freeze if there are any left over. After being frozen, they are slightly heavier and a little less crisp but still good. *Makes 6 to 8 waffles.*

Nutrients per waffle: Calories 250, Fat 11 g, Carbohydrate 34 g, Cholesterol 85 mg, Sodium 420 mg, Fiber 1 g, Protein 6 g

Crêpes

Don't be put off by the French name for these easy, make-ahead pancakes, which can be packed with various fillings to suit different tastes. They may be breakfast blintzes, fruit desserts, or a substantial brunch or luncheon main dish. Make these and freeze them to pull out anytime you want a special breakfast or brunch treat.

⅔ cup GF Mix or Four Flour Bean Mix (pages 38–39)
½ teaspoon salt
3 eggs
1½ cups milk or nondairy liquid
2 tablespoons butter, melted

Place flour, salt, and eggs in a medium bowl. Whisk together or mix with a hand beater until smooth. Slowly beat in the milk and melted butter. Place bowl in the refrigerator and let rest 1 to 2 hours.

Using a 7" skillet or crêpe pan, heat a small amount of oil and pour in ¼ cup batter, or spoon in approximately 3 tablespoons or enough for a very thin covering. You may have to tilt the pan to coat the entire bottom. Cook until the bottom of the crêpe is golden brown and the edges curl, then turn and barely cook the reverse side. Slip the crêpe onto wax paper. Repeat the process until all the batter is used. (If you have a Teflon pan, oil only for the first crêpe.) *Makes about 1 dozen 7-inch crêpes.*

The crêpes can now be frozen for later use (remember to place wax paper between them for easy separation). Or you may proceed to fill the crêpes with any desired filling.

Nutrients per crêpe: Calories 80, Fat 4 g, Carbohydrate 8 g, Cholesterol 60 mg, Sodium 140 mg, Fiber 0, Protein 3 g

Breakfast Blintzes 350°

Cheese blintzes, a Jewish-American favorite, make a wonderfully refreshing change from jam or syrup on pancakes. These can be made ahead and heated up in the oven or microwave for a treat at breakfast.

1 batch (about 12) prepared Crêpes (page 215)
1 cup cottage or ricotta cheese
One 3-ounce package cream cheese, softened
¼ cup sugar
1 teaspoon lemon juice

Preheat oven to 350°.

In a bowl, mix together the cheeses, sugar, and lemon juice.

Fill the crêpes by spooning about 1 tablespoon of the mixture into the center of each. Roll up and place seam side down in an 8″ × 12″ glass baking dish. Or you may fold the other sides in, making small packets or squares. Repeat with all 12 crêpes (or as many as you plan to make). Heat for about 15 minutes or in the microwave on medium until heated through. Serve topped with fresh or frozen and thawed fruit or berries. *Makes 1 dozen blintzes.*

Nutrients per blintz: Calories 140, Fat 8 g, Carbohydrate 13 g, Cholesterol 75 mg, Sodium 230 mg, Fiber 0, Protein 6 g

Chicken Crêpes 375°

A make-ahead dish for brunch or lunch that can be taken from the refrigerator and popped into the oven half an hour before serving time. The special flavor comes from the light ginger and curry seasonings. These go well with a combination of sliced fruits.

1 batch (about 12) prepared Crêpes (page 215)
4 tablespoons (½ stick) margarine
2 tablespoons chopped onion
2 tablespoons rice flour
½ teaspoon salt
Dash of garlic salt
1½ teaspoons sugar
2 teaspoons curry powder
½ teaspoon grated fresh ginger
1 cup chicken broth
3 cups diced cooked chicken
½ cup sour cream or nondairy substitute
2 tablespoons butter, melted

Preheat oven to 375°. Butter a 9″ × 13″ baking dish.

Melt the margarine in a large frying pan. Add the onion and sauté until tender. Stir in the rice flour, salt, garlic salt, sugar, curry, and grated ginger. Cook a minute or two, then add the broth and bring to a simmer until thickened. Add the chicken and sour cream and heat a few seconds before removing from the stove.

Place 1 or 2 heaping tablespoons of the chicken curry in the center of each crêpe. Roll the crêpe and place seam side down in the buttered dish. Repeat until the dish is full, packing them tightly. Drizzle with melted butter. Bake for 20 to 25 minutes at 375°, or until hot and bubbling. *Makes 6 servings.*

Nutrients per serving: Calories 290, Fat 21 g, Carbohydrate 14 g, Cholesterol 120 mg, Sodium 580 mg, Fiber 1 g, Protein 11 g

Florentine Crêpe Cups 350°

When I was served these by another celiac, I found them so tasty, I asked permission to put them in this book. Betty has made them with a rice mix and the bean flour. She prefers the bean flour, and so do I. To cut the cholesterol, I make mine with liquid egg substitute and nondairy creamer, but use the Cheddar cheese and mayonnaise as called for in the recipe.

CRÊPES

3 eggs, slightly beaten, or liquid egg substitute
⅔ cup Four Flour Bean Mix or GF Mix (pages 38–39)
½ teaspoon salt
1 cup milk or nondairy creamer

FILLING

3 tablespoons Four Flour Bean Mix or GF Mix
1½ cups grated sharp Cheddar cheese
3 eggs, slightly beaten, or liquid egg substitute
⅔ cup mayonnaise
One 10-ounce package frozen chopped spinach, thawed
¾ cup cooked shrimp
½ teaspoon salt

Combine the ingredients for crêpes in a blender or mixer and beat until smooth. Let stand 30 minutes.

On a hot skillet, drop 2 tablespoons of batter. Cook one side only. Put a crêpe in each of 12 muffin tins, uncooked side down.

For the filling, stir together the ingredients and fill the crêpes. Bake in a preheated 350° oven for 35 to 40 minutes, or until set. *Makes 6 servings of 2 crêpe cups each.*

Nutrients per serving: Calories 420, Fat 25 g, Carbohydrate 26 g, Cholesterol 28 mg, Sodium 880 mg, Fiber 2 g, Protein 21 g

Cranberry-Plus Coffee Cake

350°

This springy, moist coffee cake can change flavors with whatever fruit or vegetable you add to the cranberries in the recipe. I have made it successfully with chopped apples, chopped moist dried prunes, grated carrots, grated zucchini, and drained crushed pineapple. Good enough to eat as bar cookies or a square topped with whipped cream for dessert. You may substitute 1 cup Four Flour Bean Mix (pages 38–39) for the rice, soy, and potato starch flours.

2 large eggs
¾ cup sugar
⅓ cup mayonnaise
½ cup rice flour
¼ cup soy flour
¼ cup potato starch flour
½ teaspoon xanthan gum
1 teaspoon pumpkin pie spice
1 teaspoon baking powder
¼ teaspoon baking soda
1 cup fresh or frozen cranberries
1 cup chopped fruit or grated vegetable
½ cup chopped pecans, walnuts, or macadamia nuts

Preheat oven to 350°. Grease a 9″ × 9″ cake pan and dust with rice flour.

In a mixing bowl, beat together eggs, sugar, and mayonnaise.

Whisk together the flours, xanthan gum, spice, baking powder, and baking soda. Stir into the egg mixture, blending well. Stir in the whole cranberries, chopped fruit, and nuts.

Spread batter into the prepared pan. Bake at 350° until cake feels firm when touched in the center and edges begin to pull from pan, about 45 minutes. Cut into squares and serve either warm or cool. Can be made ahead and kept covered with plastic wrap for up to 3 days. *Makes 9 servings.*

Nutrients per serving: Calories 260, Fat 13 g, Carbohydrate 37 g, Cholesterol 50 mg, Sodium 135 mg, Fiber 2 g, Protein 3 g

Apple Bundt Coffee Cake 350°

The surprise is the apple filling in the center of this rich bundt cake.

1 to 2 large apples (2 cups sliced)
¼ cup apple juice
1 tablespoon cornstarch
½ teaspoon cinnamon
¼ teaspoon nutmeg
¾ cup plus 1 tablespoon sugar
⅓ cup shortening
3 eggs
½ teaspoon vanilla
1 cup sour cream or nondairy substitute
1½ cups GF Mix or Four Flour Bean Mix (pages 38–39)
½ teaspoon xanthan gum
2 teaspoons baking powder
½ teaspoon baking soda
½ teaspoon salt

Preheat oven to 350°. Grease a bundt pan and dust with rice flour.

Peel, core, and slice the apples. Place in a microwave dish and toss with the juice, cornstarch, cinnamon, and nutmeg plus the 1 tablespoon sugar. Cover with plastic wrap and microwave on High 6 to 7 minutes, stirring once or twice. (If you do not have a microwave, use ¾ cup thick applesauce, adding the cinnamon and nutmeg.) Set aside while you make the batter.

Cream ¾ cup sugar and shortening until light. Beat in the eggs and vanilla, then add the sour cream. Stir in the flour mixed with the xanthan gum, baking powder, baking soda, and salt.

Pour half the batter into the bottom of the prepared bundt pan. Over it arrange the apple mixture, keeping it from the edges of the pan. Top with the rest of the batter. Bake about 40 minutes, or until the top springs back when touched.

Unmold onto a round plate and dust the top with a bit of powdered sugar if desired. May be served warm or cold. *Makes 12 servings.*

Nutrients per serving: Calories 360, Fat 15 g, Carbohydrate 52 g, Cholesterol 90 mg, Sodium 350 mg, Fiber 1 g, Protein 4 g

Surprise Doughnut Holes

Surprise your friends with the airy lightness of these little round doughnut balls. Like all doughnuts, these are best served hot, but they still taste good cold.

1 cup water
½ cup (1 stick) butter or margarine
1 cup potato starch flour
1 tablespoon sugar
¼ teaspoon salt
4 eggs
Oil for deep-fat frying
Cinnamon sugar

In a 2-quart saucepan, heat water and butter until the mixture boils. Remove pan from heat and stir in, all at once, the combined flour, sugar, and salt. Continue stirring until the mixture forms a ball and pulls away from the sides of the pan. Then, with an electric mixer, beat in the eggs, one at a time, beating well after each addition.

Meanwhile, heat the oil for deep-fat frying. Use either an electric skillet set at 375° or an automatic deep-fry kettle (such as a Fry-Daddy). Use at least 1 inch of oil in the skillet or add oil up to the marked line on an automatic fry kettle.

Drop the batter into the heated oil by small rounded teaspoonfuls, a few at a time. Fry until they are golden brown, turning them to brown evenly. They will puff up to about 1½ inches as they cook (about 5 minutes altogether). Remove and drain on paper towels.

While still warm, shake in a plastic bag with cinnamon sugar (2 tablespoons sugar to ½ teaspoon cinnamon). *Makes 3 dozen holes.*

Nutrients per doughnut: Calories 60, Fat 4 g, Carbohydrate 5 g, Cholesterol 30 mg, Sodium 50 mg, Fiber 0, Protein 1 g

Cake Doughnuts

If you're hungry for that old-fashioned deep-fried doughnut, try this easy recipe you can make in the mixer, roll out, and cut with a doughnut cutter. Follow the recipe for an exciting orange flavor or choose the more usual variation with cinnamon and nutmeg. The texture and taste will be that of a wheat-flour doughnut.

¾ cup Garfava flour
¼ cup sorghum flour
1 cup tapioca flour
1 cup cornstarch
1½ teaspoons xanthan gum
2 teaspoons baking powder
1 teaspoon baking soda
1 teaspoon dried orange peel
Dash of salt

2 eggs
⅔ cup sugar
1 teaspoon vanilla
⅓ cup sour cream
⅓ cup orange juice concentrate, thawed
¼ cup margarine or butter, melted

In a medium bowl, whisk together the flours, cornstarch, xanthan gum, baking powder, baking soda, orange peel, and salt. Set aside.

In the bowl of your mixer, beat the eggs, sugar, and vanilla until thick and lemon-colored. Combine the sour cream, orange juice concentrate, and melted margarine. Add these alternately to the egg mixture with the dry ingredients, beating until just blended after each addition. Chill the dough for about 30 minutes.

Roll the dough out on a board dusted with sweet rice flour, working in enough sweet rice flour for the dough to be easily handled. Roll to ⅜ inch thickness and cut with a doughnut cutter. Fry in deep hot fat (375°) until golden brown (about 1 minute per side), turning once. Drain on paper towels. *Makes 2½ dozen doughnuts.*

VARIATION: For spicy doughnuts, in place of the orange peel use ½ teaspoon cinnamon and ¼ teaspoon nutmeg. Instead of the orange juice concentrate, increase the sour cream to ⅔ cup. If desired, while still warm, shake the doughnuts in a mixture of ½ cup sugar and ½ teaspoon cinnamon.

Nutrients per doughnut: Calories 80, Fat 2½ g, Carbohydrate 13 g, Cholesterol 20 mg, Sodium 130 mg, Fiber 0, Protein 1 g

Dutch Babies 425°

An oven omelet with a texture between pancake and soufflé.

¼ cup (½ stick) butter or margarine
3 eggs
½ cup milk or nondairy liquid
¼ cup GF Mix (page 38)
Powdered sugar for dusting (optional)

Melt the butter in a glass pie pan in the oven. Meanwhile, mix the eggs and milk in a blender. Add flour and blend again. Pour into pie pan. Bake 18 minutes in a preheated 425° oven. Serve with syrup, jam, or crushed fruit. Dust with powdered sugar, if desired. *Makes 4 servings.*

Nutrients per serving: Calories 210, Fat 16 g, Carbohydrate 10 g, Cholesterol 195 mg, Sodium 180 mg, Fiber 0, Protein 6 g

Vegetable Quiche with Mashed Potato Crust 350°

In my first conversation with Dr. Winkelman, he praised his wife's gluten-free quiche. Jan Winkelman shares her recipe with us here.

CRUST

3 cups mashed potatoes seasoned with salt and pepper

⅓ cup minced onion

FILLING

½ cup grated Swiss cheese

½ cup grated Cheddar cheese

½ cup sliced mushrooms

½ cup broccoli flowers

¼ cup sliced green pepper

½ cup grated carrots

3 eggs

1 cup milk

Preheat oven to 350°. Butter a 9″ pie pan.

Mix the seasoned mashed potatoes with minced onion and with them sculpt a shell in the prepared pan. Bake for 15 minutes. (Leave oven on.)

Remove from oven and layer cheeses on the bottom, then add the vegetables. Fill the crust to slightly mounded. Beat together the eggs and milk and pour over all. Bake for 30 to 40 minutes, or until you can cut through the quiche easily. *Makes 6 servings.*

VARIATION: Substitute other vegetables such as asparagus, celery, corn, and so on. For a nonvegetarian dish, add ham or cooked chicken.

VARIATION FOR THOSE ALLERGIC TO EGGS: You may substitute 1 cup liquid egg substitute for the eggs and use only ⅞ cup milk.

VARIATION FOR A RICHER QUICHE: Use either eggs or the liquid substitute with 1 cup sour cream or nondairy substitute.

Nutrients per serving: Calories 270, Fat 14 g, Carbohydrate 24 g, Cholesterol 130 mg, Sodium 540 mg, Fiber 3 g, Protein 14 g

Toad-in-the-Hole 400°

This meat and pastry dish may have been the original poor man's version of roast beef and Yorkshire pudding. A good brunch main dish, it goes well with curried fruit.

1 cup GF Mix (page 38)
2 eggs
1 cup milk or nondairy liquid
½ teaspoon salt
Pepper to taste
1 pound pork or turkey sausage links

Grease a 2-quart flat casserole.

In a food processor or blender, combine flour, eggs, milk, salt, and pepper. Mix at high speed until well blended. Refrigerate for at least 1 hour.

Meanwhile, prick each sausage with a fork and place in a frying pan with 2 tablespoons water. Cook, covered, over low heat for 2 minutes. Raise heat to medium low, uncover, and cook, turning frequently, until sausages are well browned.

Cut sausages into approximately 1-inch pieces and lay in a single layer in the casserole dish. Pour batter over them and bake in a preheated 400° oven for 30 minutes. Serve immediately. *Makes 4 to 6 servings.*

Nutrients per serving: Calories 320, Fat 18 g, Carbohydrate 24 g, Cholesterol 120 mg, Sodium 730 mg, Fiber 0, Protein 16 g

Overnight Casserole 350°

A hearty brunch or luncheon casserole that goes from the refrigerator to the oven, saving the busy hostess time in the morning to get ready for guests.

6 to 8 slices GF bread, crusts removed
6 slices Swiss cheese
1 pound ground pork sausage (see Note)
6 eggs
2 cups milk or nondairy liquid
Dash of salt

Line a 9″ × 13″ greased pan with enough bread to cover the bottom. Top with slices of Swiss cheese and the pork sausage, which has been cooked a little and drained.

Beat the eggs and add the milk and salt. Pour this mixture over the bread and refrigerate overnight. Bake the next morning in a preheated 350° oven for 1 hour. *Makes 6 servings.*

NOTE: Ground turkey may be substituted for the pork sausage. Be sure to season the turkey well. GF sausage seasoning can be purchased from some meat markets. The usual ratio is 2 teaspoons seasoning per pound of ground meat.

Nutrients per serving: Calories 500, Fat 31 g, Carbohydrate 27 g, Cholesterol 305 mg, Sodium 1160 mg, Fiber 1 g, Protein 28 g

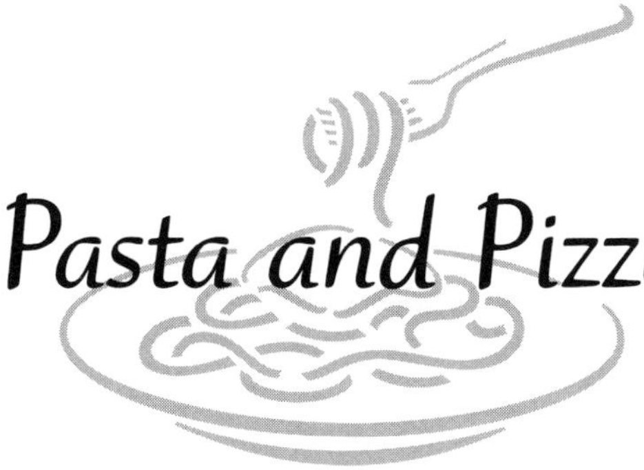

Pasta and Pizza

There is no more need for the celiac to watch other people eat pasta while he or she pushes rice around under the spaghetti sauce. I know it's not the same, for I tried that before I discovered that some dietary food companies produce gluten-free spaghetti, macaroni, and other pastas. (See pages 309–15 for listing.) You can also purchase rice noodles and bean threads in the Asian section of most grocery stores. Corn and brown rice pastas can be found in some supermarkets and health food stores. Although these are blander than homemade pasta, they will satisfy a pasta craving, especially if you cook the pasta in a beef-flavored stock or flavor it with a lot of cheese.

But other pasta dishes, such as lasagne, stroganoff, and chicken and noodles, seem to need old-fashioned, homemade egg noodles. I finally developed a recipe using gluten-free flours that satisfies my taste in these dishes—and also that of my nonceliac pasta-loving friends. With the introduction of bean flours I've discovered they make an even more exciting pasta with a great taste. They even handle better. The pastas in the following recipes work well in a pasta machine, but you don't have to have one, even for ravioli. I give directions for making all the pastas without a machine. If you have one, follow the manufacturer's directions.

As for pizza, you don't have to curb your desire for that dish. I include recipes for four tasty crusts. Just use your imagination on the topping and have pizza anytime you crave it.

Pasta and Pasta Dishes

Homemade Pasta

The following pasta is the result of much experimentation. The mixture of the many flours plus the xanthan gum seems to be the secret of success. This makes a small recipe, so you can use it immediately or freeze the uncooked pasta to cook later. The recipe may be doubled and worked in 2 balls instead of 1 for more servings.

⅓ cup tapioca flour
2 tablespoons potato starch flour
⅓ cup cornstarch
½ teaspoon salt
1 tablespoon xanthan gum
2 large eggs
1 tablespoon vegetable oil

Combine flours, cornstarch, salt, and xanthan gum. Beat eggs lightly and add oil. Pour egg into flour mixture and stir. This will feel much like pastry dough. Work together into a firm ball. Knead a minute or two.

Place ball of dough on your bread board dusted with cornstarch and roll *as thin as possible.* One pasta book suggests you should be able to see the board through the dough. The dough is tough and, although almost transparent, will still handle well. Slice the noodles into very thin strips or, if using for lasagne, into 1½ × 4-inch rectangles. The pasta is now ready to cook, or to freeze uncooked for later use.

Cook the pasta in salted boiling water to which 1 tablespoon of oil has been added for 10 to 20 minutes, depending on the thickness and the size of your pieces. You will have to test for doneness. *Makes 3 servings as noodles alone, 5 to 6 servings in a mixed casserole.*

Nutrients per serving: Calories 110, Fat 4 g, Carbohydrate 16 g, Cholesterol 70 mg, Sodium 210 mg, Fiber 1 g, Protein 2 g

After years of abstinence, probably the first thing you will want to do is eat the noodles hot from the pan, slathered with butter and grated Parmesan cheese.

Use either of these pastas in all the following pasta recipes, whether cut in thin noodles, wide lasagne strips, spaghetti, or even in the ravioli recipe.

SPAGHETTI: Use the spaghetti cutter on your pasta machine. If you don't have a pasta machine, roll the dough very thin and cut your spaghetti as narrow as possible. This may turn out a bit uneven, but no one will notice when it is hidden under spaghetti sauce. Cook for 10 minutes in boiling salted water to which a tablespoon of oil has been added.

CHOW MEIN NOODLES: Make the pasta and cut as if for spaghetti. Then cut these strips into 1- to 1½-inch pieces. Drop uncooked into hot oil and cook for a few seconds (they will probably take less than a minute). Remove from oil and drain on paper towels. Use immediately or freeze. *Makes about 5 to 6 cups chow mein noodles.*

Green Pasta Made with Broccoli

This is similar to pasta made with spinach; I think it has a better flavor.

¼ cup cooked broccoli
⅓ cup tapioca flour
¼ cup potato starch flour
⅓ cup cornstarch
½ teaspoon salt
1 tablespoon xanthan gum
2 large eggs
1 tablespoon vegetable oil

Pat the broccoli as dry as possible with paper toweling. Purée it in blender.

Combine the flours (reserving 1 tablespoon of the potato starch flour), cornstarch, salt, and xanthan gum. Stir in the broccoli. Beat eggs and oil together. Add to the flours and work into a firm ball. Add the extra tablespoon of potato starch flour if needed to make the dough dry enough to handle and roll out.

Place ball of dough on a cornstarch-dusted board and roll out as thin as possible. Cut the noodles into thin strips. You are now ready to cook these or freeze them for later use.

Suggestions for serving: Boil the noodles in salted water until done. Drain, but leave them in the saucepan on stove turned to low. Add 2 tablespoons butter, about ¼ cup cream, and ¾ cup grated Cheddar cheese. Stir until the cheese melts. Swirl onto an oval platter. *Makes 3 or 4 servings.*

Nutrients per serving: Calories 180, Fat 6 g, Carbohydrate 28 g, Cholesterol 105 mg, Sodium 320 mg, Fiber 1 g, Protein 4 g

Bean Flour Pasta

Since I discovered bean flour for cooking, I've found that it makes not only cakes and breads but a wonderfully nutty-tasting pasta. It's easy to roll out, cut, and cook. I prefer the liquid egg substitute in this, not only to cut cholesterol but to make the rolling out easier.

⅓ cup Garfava flour
⅓ cup tapioca flour
⅓ cup cornstarch
2 teaspoons xanthan gum
½ teaspoon salt
1 tablespoon vegetable or olive oil
½ cup liquid egg substitute or 2 eggs
Cornstarch for kneading

In a medium bowl, combine the flours, cornstarch, xanthan gum, and salt. Whisk together the oil and egg substitute. Pour into the flours and stir until a ball forms. Knead a minute or two, adding more cornstarch if necessary. Work it in until the dough will not accept any more and is firm and dry enough to roll.

Place the ball on a cutting board dusted with cornstarch and roll as thin as possible. It should be stretchy and elastic but roll out very thin and handle easily. Slice into very narrow strips for spaghetti, wider ones for noodles or fettuccine. If using for lasagne, cut into 1½ × 5- or 6-inch rectangles. The pasta is ready to cook immediately or to freeze uncooked for later use.

If you have a hand-crank machine (Atlas or other make), the dough can be flattened and cut with that.

To cook, drop into boiling salted water to which a few drops of oil have been added. The cooking will take from 5 to 7 minutes, depending on whether the pasta is to be used for a casserole (leave al dente) or eaten with cheese or sauce. You will have to test for doneness. *Makes 3 to 4 servings for fettuccine, enough for the Three-Cheese Lasagne (page 238), or 5 to 6 servings of a noodle casserole.*

Nutrients per serving: Calories 130, Fat 4 g, Carbohydrate 20 g, Cholesterol 70 mg, Sodium 200 mg, Fiber 0 g, Protein 4 g

Easy Fettuccine

This is a light version of fettuccine.

1 recipe Homemade Pasta, (page 230), cut into ⅛-inch strips
¼ cup ricotta cheese
¼ cup plain yogurt
¼ cup grated Parmesan cheese
1 tablespoon margarine
Dash of black pepper

Cook the pasta in salted water. Drain well and return to the cooking pot. Add the ricotta cheese, yogurt, Parmesan cheese, margarine, and pepper and toss well to mix.

Transfer to a warm platter and serve. *Makes 3 servings.*

Nutrients per serving: Calories 230, Fat 13 g, Carbohydrate 18 g, Cholesterol 50 mg, Sodium 450 mg, Fiber 1 g, Protein 9 g

Fettuccine Alfredo (Lightened)

I've cut some of the extra calories from this usually high-fat sauce. Use this on your purchased or homemade pastas. It goes especially well with the Bean Flour Pasta (page 232). Regular curly parsley may be substituted for the cilantro.

8 ounces purchased GF pasta or 1 recipe Homemade Pasta (page 230)
1⅓ cups milk or nondairy substitute
2 tablespoons GF Mix (page 38)
1 clove garlic, minced
⅓ cup grated Romano cheese
Pinch nutmeg
¼ teaspoon salt
¼ teaspoon pepper
2 teaspoons butter or margarine
¼ cup chopped cilantro
¼ cup grated Parmesan cheese
Fresh parsley for garnish (optional)

Start the pasta cooking according to directions.

Meanwhile, in a medium saucepan, whisk the milk and flour together. Add the garlic and cook over medium heat, stirring often, until the mixture becomes slightly thickened. Add the Romano cheese, nutmeg, salt, and pepper. Stir until the cheese melts.

Drain the pasta and transfer to a bowl. Toss with the butter and cilantro. Stir in the cheese sauce and toss again. Spoon into 4 serving dishes or onto plates and sprinkle each serving with the Parmesan cheese. Garnish with the parsley sprigs, if desired. *Makes 4 servings.*

Nutrients per serving: Calories 146, Fat 6 g, Carbohydrate 19 g, Cholesterol 92 mg, Sodium 312 mg, Fiber 1 g, Protein 3 g

Pasta Provolone

A richer, cheesier dish than the preceding ones.

1 recipe Homemade Pasta, (page 230), cut in thin strips
1½ cups grated Monterey Jack cheese
1 cup grated provolone cheese
½ cup cream or nondairy substitute
1 cup sliced pitted ripe olives
1 tomato, cut in thin wedges
2 tablespoons dried basil
¼ cup pine nuts

In a large saucepan, cook the pasta. Drain and return the pasta to the dry pan. Add the cheeses and cream and heat, stirring to melt the cheese. Stir in the olives, tomato, basil, and pine nuts. Heat through and serve immediately. *Makes 4 or 5 servings.*

Nutrients per serving: Calories 350, Fat 30 g, Carbohydrate 9 g, Cholesterol 70 mg, Sodium 610 mg, Fiber 2 g, Protein 18 g

Ham and Chicken Pasta

Another of those melt-in-the-mouth noodle dishes. My favorite.

1 recipe Homemade Pasta, (page 230), cut into ⅛-inch strips
4 egg yolks
1 cup cream or nondairy substitute
4 tablespoons (½ stick) butter
½ cup chicken or turkey strips
½ cup ham strips
Salt and pepper to taste
1 cup grated Parmesan cheese

Cook the pasta and drain.

In a small bowl, blend egg yolks and cream together.

Place butter in a skillet and melt. Add the chicken and ham to brown lightly, then add the cooked pasta. Heat through. Add the egg yolks and cream and gently fold in until all is well mixed. Season to taste with salt and pepper before stirring in the grated cheese.

Serve immediately. *Makes 4 or 5 servings.*

Nutrients per serving: Calories 450, Fat 32 g, Carbohydrate 22 g, Cholesterol 300 mg, Sodium 990 mg, Fiber 1 g, Protein 20 g

Meat Sauce for Spaghetti

This is a rich, tasty sauce.

1 pound lean ground beef
¼ cup chopped onion
2 cloves garlic, minced
¼ cup chopped parsley
¼ teaspoon basil
¼ teaspoon thyme
¼ teaspoon marjoram
One 8-ounce can sliced mushrooms
One 16-ounce can tomatoes
Two 8-ounce cans tomato sauce
Pinch each allspice, cloves, and nutmeg
½ teaspoon salt
Pepper to taste

Cook meat until brown with onion and garlic. Add chopped parsley, basil, thyme, marjoram, mushrooms, canned tomatoes, and tomato sauce. Add spices and salt and pepper. Bring to a boil, turn down the heat, and simmer for at least 2 hours. Serve over GF spaghetti. *Makes 6 servings.*

EASY VARIATION: Many of the commercial spaghetti sauces on the market are gluten free, so you can use them as they come from the jar or you can brown 1 pound of lean ground beef and 1 diced onion in skillet, add salt and pepper to taste, and then pour in 1 jar (approximately 26 ounces) of your favorite GF spaghetti sauce. Bring to a boil, turn down the heat, cover, and let simmer for 2 hours for the flavors to meld. Serve over cooked GF spaghetti and top, if desired, with grated Parmesan cheese.

Nutrients per serving: Calories 230, Fat 12 g, Carbohydrate 12 g, Cholesterol 40 mg, Sodium 860 mg, Fiber 2 g, Protein 17 g

Three-Cheese Lasagne 350°

Lasagne so good that when I took this to a lasagne party, my dish was the first one emptied. I cut lasagne noodles with a pastry cutter to give a slightly wavy edge to the pasta.

1 recipe Homemade Pasta, (page 230), cut into 1½ × 4-inch rectangles
1 pound extra-lean ground beef
12 ounces mozzarella cheese
4 ounces Cheddar cheese
1 egg
One 16-ounce carton ricotta cheese
One 16-ounce jar GF spaghetti sauce

Preheat oven to 350°

While the pasta is cooking in salted water with a bit of oil added, brown the meat in a heavy frying pan, and grate the mozzarella and Cheddar cheeses. Add the egg to the ricotta and blend together.

Now assemble the ingredients in a shallow casserole approximately 9″ × 13″. Pour a little sauce on the bottom and on it place a layer of cooked noodles, using one-third of your noodles. Over this spread half the ricotta mixture, half the meat, and half the mozzarella. Spread on about one-third of the sauce. Layer another row of pasta and repeat. Top with pasta, the remaining sauce, and the grated Cheddar cheese.

Bake until the sauce bubbles around the edges, about 30 minutes.

This can be made ahead and baked just before serving, or it can be frozen before or after baking. I usually make two casseroles and we eat one fresh; I freeze the other unbaked for another meal. If you store it, frozen or unfrozen, cover it with plastic wrap, not aluminum foil. Foil can react with the tomato sauce, shedding gray flakes over the lasagne. *Serves 6 to 10,* depending on how much else is served with it.

Nutrients per serving: Calories 450, Fat 30 g, Carbohydrate 20 g, Cholesterol 165 mg, Sodium 650 mg, Fiber 1 g, Protein 26 g

VEGETARIAN LASAGNE: Omit the meat and increase the Cheddar to 12 ounces. Mix the Cheddar with the mozzarella as you make the layers. If you wish, you may sauté about 1 cup of sliced mushrooms in butter and add them to the layers or add 1 well-drained 10-ounce package of thawed spinach.

MOCK LASAGNE: Here is a lasagne without noodles, using instead one package (6 to 8) thick corn tortillas. Slice the tortillas into strips about 1½ inches wide and layer with the remaining ingredients from either of the two preceding lasagne recipes. If you bake it immediately, the lasagne will have a mild corn taste. But if this is frozen and later thawed and baked, the flavor will be more like that of conventional lasagne.

Three-Cheese Ravioli

This simple three-cheese filling is one of the easiest to make and handle. This makes enough for a triple batch of pasta.

¾ cup ricotta cheese
2 tablespoons grated sharp Cheddar
2 tablespoons grated mozzarella
Salt and pepper to taste
1 small egg plus 1 egg reserved for wash
Triple recipe Homemade Pasta (page 230) or Bean Flour Pasta (page 232)

Blend cheeses, salt and pepper, and 1 egg in food processor until creamy.

Prepare the pasta. If you have a pasta machine with the ravioli attachment, follow directions for filling and cutting. If you have the inexpensive ravioli tray, follow directions for using it.

If you have neither, roll the sheet of pasta out to about 12 × 14 inches. Paint one side with a wash of beaten egg mixed with a little water. Onto this, drop the cheese filling in dabs less than ½ inch in size from the tip of a teaspoon. They should be about 2 to 2¼ inches apart. When the side is filled, fold the dough over and, with fingers or a rounded spoon handle, seal the dough between the small mounds. Cut with a pastry cutter or use a product called Krimpkut Sealer specially made for cutting and sealing at the same time. You should work quickly so the egg wash stays moist to help the pasta seal. Repeat with remaining pasta. When the ravioli are all made, either cook immediately in a large pot of boiling, salted water for 15 minutes (test for doneness) or freeze for later use. *Makes about 90 ravioli, or 10 to 12 servings.*

These are excellent served with a meat sauce (page 237).

Nutrients per serving: Calories 70, Fat 4 g, Carbohydrate 4 g, Cholesterol 60 mg, Sodium 115 mg, Fiber 0, Protein 4 g

Chicken Ravioli

A delicately flavored ravioli in a creamy white sauce, different and good.

FILLING

¼ cup cooked broccoli
¾ cup cooked chicken
2 tablespoons grated Cheddar cheese
Salt and pepper to taste
1 small egg
2 or 3 tablespoons chicken broth

Triple recipe Homemade Pasta (page 230) or Bean Flour Pasta (page 232)

SAUCE

4 tablespoons (½ stick) butter
2 tablespoons sweet rice flour
2 cups cream or nondairy substitute
⅓ teaspoon nutmeg
Dash of pepper
⅔ cup grated Cheddar cheese

Put all filling ingredients except the chicken broth in the blender or food processor. Blend them. Add the chicken broth a little at a time, blending after each addition, until filling has a creamy consistency.

Make a triple batch of pasta and follow the directions on pages 239–40 for completing the ravioli. Freeze for later use or cook for 15 minutes in salted water. Test for doneness. Serve hot with the sauce.

Melt the butter in a 2-quart saucepan on medium-low heat. Add the rice flour, stir, and slowly add the cream, continuing to stir so it doesn't lump. Add the nutmeg and pepper and continue to stir as the sauce thickens slightly. Add the cheese and blend in until it melts. The sauce is now ready to serve. Either put the ravioli into the sauce or pour the sauce over the hot ravioli in the serving dish. (I like to use a large low dish.) Sprinkle the top with nutmeg or paprika. *Makes 12 servings.*

Nutrients per serving: Calories 180, Fat 12 g, Carbohydrate 10 g, Cholesterol 60 mg, Sodium 400 mg, Fiber 0, Protein 6 g

Chicken Noodle Casserole 350°

An old favorite with a new taste.

1 recipe Homemade Pasta (page 230) or Bean Flour Pasta (page 232), cut into ¼-inch strips
2 cups diced cooked chicken
One recipe Creamed Soup Base (cooked) (page 292)
One 3-ounce package cream cheese
½ cup chicken broth
1 teaspoon poultry seasoning
3 green onions, thinly sliced
One 8-ounce can water chestnuts, drained and sliced
4 ounces sliced almonds

Make pasta, cut, and cook. If you add 2 tablespoons of powdered chicken soup base to the noodle water, the noodles will have more flavor. Drain and rinse pasta.

Place chicken and noodles in a large casserole. Blend the cream cheese with the cooked cream soup and thin with chicken broth. Stir in the poultry seasoning, green onions, and water chestnuts. Spread this mixture over the chicken and noodles. You may fold the sliced almonds into the mixture or scatter them on top of the assembled casserole.

Bake in preheated 350° oven for 45 to 50 minutes. *Makes 6 servings.*

Nutrients per serving: Calories 370, Fat 20 g, Carbohydrate 21 g, Cholesterol 90 mg, Sodium 323 mg, Fiber 4 g, Protein 27 g

Tuna-Cashew Casserole 325°

I pulled this old standby out of my recipe file and found it excellent with chow mein noodles.

One recipe mushroom Creamed Soup Base (page 292)
1¼ cups milk or nondairy liquid
3½ cups cooked Chow Mein Noodles (page 231)
One 6½-ounce can tuna fish
⅓ cup cashew nuts
1 cup diced celery
¼ cup minced onion
Dash of pepper
Salt to taste

Mix mushroom soup and milk and pour over the remaining ingredients, which have been placed in a 2-quart casserole. Stir together to moisten thoroughly. Bake in a preheated 325° oven for 50 to 60 minutes. *Makes 6 to 8 servings.*

Nutrients per serving: Calories 360, Fat 26 g, Carbohydrate 21 g, Cholesterol 30 mg, Sodium 640 mg, Fiber 4 g, Protein 25 g

Beef Stroganoff

For years I envied my husband being able to order beef stroganoff in restaurants while I could only watch him eat it. After I created the recipe for homemade pasta, I worked on the stroganoff recipe and came up with this easy, excellent dish. I make the pasta and let it dry a bit while preparing the sauce. Then, after adding the sour cream, I cook the pasta while the sauce is heating.

1 pound beef sirloin
3 tablespoons rice flour
½ teaspoon salt
2 tablespoons vegetable oil
One 3-ounce can sliced mushrooms, or ½ cup sliced fresh mushrooms
1 cup chopped onion
1 clove garlic, minced
1 tablespoon ketchup
1 can beef broth, or 1¼ cups instant beef stock
1 cup sour cream or nondairy substitute
2 tablespoons rice wine or dry white wine
1 recipe Homemade Pasta, (page 230) or Bean Flour Pasta (page 232), cut into noodles

Cut beef into ¼-inch strips. Combine 1 tablespoon flour and salt and coat the meat. Heat a skillet, add the oil, and drop in coated meat. Brown quickly. Add drained canned or sliced fresh mushrooms, onion, and garlic. Cook 3 or 4 minutes, until onion is crisp but tender.

Remove meat and mushrooms from pan. Add a bit more oil to pan drippings and blend in 2 remaining tablespoons flour. Put ketchup in beef broth and stir into pan. Cook, stirring, over medium heat until thickened and bubbly.

Return browned meat and mushrooms to skillet. Stir in sour cream and wine. Cook slowly until heated through. Do not boil. Keep warm over hot water while you cook the pasta. Serve sauce over hot buttered noodles. *Makes 4 or 5 servings.*

Nutrients per serving: Calories 550, Fat 29 g, Carbohydrate 37 g, Cholesterol 185 mg, Sodium 1070 mg, Fiber 2 g, Protein 34 g

Pizzas

Pat's Thin Yeast Crust

425°

Pat Garst, author of Gluten-Free Cooking, *shares this recipe for a thin yeast crust for pizza. This is easy to make, with great flavor.*

1½ teaspoons instant dry yeast granules
About 1 cup warm water, 105° to 115°
1 teaspoon sugar
⅔ cup rice flour
⅓ cup potato starch flour
1 tablespoon potato flour
1½ teaspoons melted shortening
1 teaspoon salt

Preheat oven to 425°.

In a mixing bowl, dissolve the yeast in ½ cup of the warm water with the sugar added. Let set until yeast bubbles and the quantity doubles.

Add all the rest of the ingredients, using enough of the remaining water to get a dough the consistency of cake frosting that will spread, not run, when all ingredients are thoroughly beaten. Grease a 10″ × 15″ jelly roll pan. Pour batter down the center and spread with a spatula. Run a teaspoon around the edges, forcing batter up the sides.

If you prefer, you may do as I do and pour the batter and spread in a circle on the pan, forming a 12- to 12½-inch circle with raised edges. The batter handles well and will make a circle shape easily. Leave more at edges for raised sides.

You may fill immediately with the sauce (see page 248) and toppings or, for a crisp Sicilian-type crust, bake for 10 minutes and then top and return to the oven for 25 to 30 minutes. *Makes 6 to 8 servings.*

Nutrients per serving: Calories 110, Fat 1.5 g, Carbohydrate 24 g, Cholesterol 0, Sodium 380 mg, Fiber 1 g, Protein 2 g

Jill's Quick and Easy Pizza Crust

400°

Jill Ryan claims she never makes anything unless it can be quick and easy. This is especially true for her excellent pizza crust recipe.

¼ cup milk
2 large eggs
⅓ cup cornstarch
⅔ cup rice flour
¼ teaspoon xanthan gum
1 teaspoon salt
¼ cup shortening, melted

Beat the milk and eggs together. Add the cornstarch, flour, xanthan gum, and salt. Mix in melted shortening.

Spread into a greased 9″ × 13″ pan or (as I do) spread with a spatula in a 12-inch circle about ¼ inch thick on a cookie sheet or round pizza pan, leaving a thicker crust around the outside of the circle to keep the sauce and cheese from running over onto the pan.

Spread sauce evenly over the unbaked crust and top with your favorite toppings (see page 248). Bake in preheated 400° oven for about 25 minutes. *Makes 6 servings.*

Nutrients per serving: Calories 200, Fat 11 g, Carbohydrate 21 g, Cholesterol 75 mg, Sodium 410 mg, Fiber 0, Protein 3 g

Thick Yeast-free Pizza Crust

400°

For a thicker pizza crust, try this easy recipe, which requires no rising but tastes like a yeast bread crust.

1 cup potato starch flour
½ cup tapioca flour
½ cup cornstarch
½ cup dry milk powder
1 tablespoon baking powder
½ teaspoon salt
2 tablespoons shortening
¾ cup water

Preheat oven to 400°.

In a mixing bowl, place the flours, cornstarch, dry milk, baking powder, and salt. Cut in the shortening, rubbing with the fingers until it feels like cornmeal. Pour in the water and stir until the dough clings together in a ball. Work with the hands, kneading the dough until smooth. Form into 2 balls.

Place a ball in the center of a greased cookie sheet or pizza tin, cover it with plastic wrap, and press it out into a 10-inch circle about ¼ inch thick except at the edges, which should be about ½ inch thick to contain the sauce and fillings. Repeat with the second ball. Fill with desired sauce and toppings (see page 248). Bake for 20 to 22 minutes.

To freeze one of the pizzas, place it on a prepared, foil-covered cardboard circle and fill as above. Wrap securely with plastic wrap, then foil, and place in freezer. To cook, slide from the wrappings to the cookie sheet without thawing and bake a few minutes longer than the specified time. If defrosted first, use the cooking time above. *Each pizza will make 6 servings.*

Nutrients per serving: Calories 250, Fat 7 g, Carbohydrate 44 g, Cholesterol 10 mg, Sodium 300 mg, Fiber 0, Protein 3 g

Yeast-Rising Thick Pizza Crust

400°

This is it, the yeast-rising thick pizza crust you've been hungering for. This is simple to make, freezes well, and will fool your friends into thinking they are eating pizza with a wheat crust.

2 cups rice flour
2 cups tapioca flour
⅔ cup dry milk powder or nondairy substitute
3½ teaspoons xanthan gum
1 teaspoon salt
2 teaspoons pizza seasoning (optional)
2 tablespoons dry yeast granules
1 cup lukewarm water, 105° to 115°
1 tablespoon sugar
3 tablespoons shortening
½ cup hot water
4 egg whites, at room temperature

In the bowl of a heavy-duty mixer, put flours, milk, xanthan gum, and salt. Dissolve the yeast in the lukewarm water with the tablespoon of sugar added. Melt the shortening in the hot water.

With the mixer on low, blend the dry ingredients adding the seasoning, if desired. Pour in the hot water and shortening, blending to mix. Add the egg whites, blend again, then add the yeast mixture. Beat on high speed for 4 minutes.

Spoon half the dough onto a greased cookie sheet or round pizza tin. With your hand in a plastic bag, pat the dough out in a circle about ¼ inch thick except at the edges, which should be higher to contain the sauce and fillings. Repeat with the second half of the dough.

Let rise 10 minutes, then bake in preheated 400° oven 5 to 7 minutes before spreading with your sauce and favorite toppings (see page 248). Bake 20 to 22 minutes more. *Makes two 12½-inch pizzas serving 8 to 12.*

Nutrients per serving: Calories 240, Fat 5 g, Carbohydrate 42 g, Cholesterol 5 mg, Sodium 240 mg, Fiber 1 g, Protein 5 g

Pizza Sauce and Toppings

There are gluten-free pizza sauces on the market, or you can make your own using this recipe from Jill Ryan.

One 8-ounce can tomato sauce
½ teaspoon crushed oregano leaves
Garlic powder
½ teaspoon dried crushed basil
2 tablespoons sugar (or to taste)

Mix the above ingredients and spread them evenly over any 12-inch unbaked crust. Top with the following or anything you desire:

1 cup or more shredded mozzarella cheese
1 pound ground pork sausage, cooked in small chunks and drained
One 2¼-ounce can sliced olives, drained
Sliced fresh mushrooms (optional)

Other toppings could include sardines, sliced salami, sliced green peppers, minced ham, a second cheese, or other items of your choice.

Nutrients per serving: Calories 20, Fat 0, Carbohydrate 5 g, Cholesterol 0, Sodium 170 mg, Fiber 0, Protein 0

Minipizza Tricks

For a quick minipizza for a single serving try topping a thick corn tortilla with sauce and toppings. Bake in a preheated 375° oven for approximately 12 minutes.

Another minipizza can be made for one person or enough for a crowd of hungry teenagers by slicing English Muffins (see page 211) and topping with sauce and cheese. Bake as above.

Appetizers and Snacks

See Also

Trying to snack from a party table is usually frustrating to a celiac or anyone who must avoid wheat.

Some cheeses contain flavorings that are not gluten free, and many prepared meat slices use wheat starch for a binder. Beware of dips that might contain gluten in their seasonings, and avoid any cream mixtures whose base is questionable. Crackers or buns will usually have a wheat flour base.

Thus, the celiac must stick to eating only the cheeses he or she is familiar with, the raw vegetables, the potato chips, and the wheat-free corn chips. (Some flavored chips may contain gluten in the seasoning.)

If you know you are going to attend a function where only appetizers and dips will be served, you might carry your own rice crackers, which you can find in the Asian section of most large grocery stores, or, if possible, suggest to the hostess that you make and bring one of the dishes. There are several packaged salad dressing mixes that are gluten free and may be safely combined with mayonnaise and sour cream as a dip for raw vegetables or potato chips. For a dip lower in calories, replace the sour cream with cottage cheese. Any hostess would be happy to have this addition to her table.

I've included here a few more elaborate family favorites and some created by my friends when they were challenged by my diet. I've also added a granola mix great for munching, as a cereal at breakfast, as a snack on a trail hike, or made up into bars by the recipe included.

You'll find other appetizers in the Holiday Fare chapter.

Cheese Ball

Purchased cheese balls are often made with a seasoning or filler containing gluten, so why not make your own? This simple recipe takes only a short time to prepare and can be made ahead of time and refrigerated.

½ cup grated Cheddar cheese
One 8-ounce package cream cheese
¼ cup mayonnaise
½ cup minced onion
Dash of salt (or to taste)
¼ cup finely chopped pecan meats

Blend both cheeses, mayonnaise, onion, and salt. Shape into a ball and place in refrigerator until firm. Roll ball in nuts. Store in refrigerator. Serve with small rice crackers at the side and let people spread from the ball onto their crackers. *Makes a ball about 2½ inches in diameter. Makes 16 servings.*

Nutrients per serving: Calories 110, Fat 9 g, Carbohydrate 4 g, Cholesterol 25 mg, Sodium 190 mg, Fiber 0, Protein 2 g

Shrimp Cheese Spread

This hors d'oeuvre served hot from the broiler makes your guests think you've gone to a lot of trouble for them. But don't save it just for guests. Use it for late-evening snacking or let it take the place of other munchies while watching afternoon games on television.

8 ounces sharp cheese
One 4-ounce can shrimp, drained
3 green onions
¼ green pepper
One 8-ounce can ripe olives, drained
½ cup (1 stick) margarine, melted
One 8-ounce can tomato sauce

Grind together or blend in food processor the cheese, shrimp, green onions, green pepper, and pitted olives. Then add the melted margarine and the tomato sauce.

Spread this mixture on split GF buns or slices of GF bread. These may be cut into circles with a biscuit cutter or (as I prefer) into triangles, 2 or 4 to a slice, depending on how fancy your party. Put them under the broiler until the spread melts and bubbles. The mixture will keep several days in the refrigerator, and the buns or bread can be spread shortly ahead of time. *Makes approximately 1½ pints, serving 8 to 12.*

Nutrients per serving: Calories 170, Fat 16 g, Carbohydrate 3 g, Cholesterol 55 mg, Sodium 870 mg, Fiber 1 g, Protein 7 g

Ham and Cheese Spread

This quick and easy spread will make even rice crackers taste good, but it is especially tasty on toasted or dried triangles of some of the pumpernickel or bean bread slices.

One 8-ounce package cream cheese (regular or ⅓ fat reduced), softened
One 4.75-ounce can honey ham spread or deviled ham
½ cup crushed pineapple, drained well
2 green onions, thinly sliced
1 tablespoon mayonnaise (optional)

In a medium bowl, combine the cream cheese and ham spread. Beat until smooth. Add the pineapple and green onions, mixing well. For a more spreadable consistency, add the mayonnaise, if desired. Refrigerate for 30 minutes or until serving. (May be made a day ahead.) *Makes 2 cups. Serving size: 1 tablespoon.*

Nutrients per serving: Calories 970, Fat 77 g, Carbohydrate 37 g, Cholesterol 220 mg, Sodium 261 mg, Fiber 1 g, Protein 36 g

Cheese Sticks

400°

If you're tired of the same gluten-free crackers on the grocery shelves, try baking your own. These cheese sticks are great for parties, but they also taste good with soups, in lunches, or for just plain snacking. Their flavor varies with the strength of the cheese; I use medium Cheddar, but if you love sharp cheese, use that.

8 ounces Cheddar cheese
2 tablespoons butter or margarine
1 large egg
½ teaspoon salt
⅛ teaspoon ground pepper
¾ cup rice flour
¼ cup potato starch flour
1 teaspoon xanthan gum

Preheat oven to 400°

Grate the cheese (you should have approximately 2 cups). Set aside. Place butter in bowl of mixer and beat until creamy. Add egg, salt, and pepper. Beat until blended. Beat in cheese one-third at a time until combined. Stir in flours and xanthan gum until thoroughly blended. Work the dough into a ball. If dough doesn't stick together, add cold water, 1 tablespoon at a time, until a ball can be formed. Don't worry about overworking. The sticks can be firm.

Divide dough, rolling half at a time between sheets of wax paper or plastic wrap to form a 7 × 14-inch rectangle about ⅛ inch thick. Cut with a pastry wheel into ½ × 7-inch strips and place on baking sheets. Bake for 6 to 8 minutes, until deep golden.

Let cool on racks and store airtight up to 1 week. *Makes 56 cheese sticks.*

Nutrients per stick: Calories 25, Fat 1 g, Carbohydrate 2 g, Cholesterol 5 mg, Sodium 55 mg, Fiber 0, Protein 1 g

CHEESE NIPS: After dividing the dough, place 1 ball on a baking sheet, cover with plastic wrap, and roll as thin as possible. Repeat with the other half. Sprinkle with salt, if desired, and cut with a pastry wheel into 1-inch squares. Bake for 4 to 6 minutes, until deep golden. *Makes about 12 dozen Nips.*

Nutrients per cracker: Calories 10, Fat ½ g, Carbohydrate 1 g, Cholesterol 5 mg, Sodium 20 mg, Fiber 0, Protein 0

Pups in Blankets

400°

Prepare pastry for Cheese Sticks, using medium-sharp Cheddar cheese. Roll out as described but cut into 1- × 4-inch bars. On each, place cut sections of small gluten-free hot dogs or cocktail sausages. Roll the pastry around the meat. Bake in preheated 400° oven for 6 to 8 minutes. These can be prepared ahead of time and popped into the oven just before serving. Makes about 4 dozen pups in blankets.

Cheese Puffs   400°

This chou pastry is far easier to make than your guests will think. These tiny puffs will elicit raves. If you wish, you may use ½ cup potato starch flour and ½ cup rice flour instead of all potato starch flour.

4 ounces Cheddar cheese
1 cup water
½ cup (1 stick) margarine or butter
⅛ teaspoon nutmeg
1 cup potato starch flour
4 large eggs

Preheat oven to 400°.

Grate the cheese (you should have 1 cup). Set aside. Place water, margarine, and nutmeg in a 2- to 3-quart saucepan. Bring to a full boil over medium heat. Turn off the heat and add the flour all at once, stirring until mixture leaves sides of pan and forms a ball. Remove from stove.

Add eggs, one at a time, beating well after each addition. Stir in ½ cup of the grated cheese. Drop the mixture by small spoonfuls on a greased baking sheet to make balls about 1½ inches in diameter. Sprinkle remaining cheese on puffs.

Bake at 400° for 20 to 25 minutes, until golden brown. Remove baking sheet from oven. Prick the puffs with a fork and return to turned-off oven for 5 minutes to crisp. Serve warm. *Makes about 3 dozen puffs.*

Nutrients per puff: Calories 60, Fat 4 g, Carbohydrate 4 g, Cholesterol 35 mg, Sodium 85 mg, Fiber 0, Protein 1 g

Mushroom Tarts 350°

These bite-sized appetizers can be made ahead and frozen, to be pulled out and reheated in the microwave while the party is in progress. The compliments you get from guests will prove they are well worth the trouble.

PASTRY DOUGH

3 ounces cream cheese, at room temperature
½ cup (1 stick) butter or margarine
⅓ cup rice flour
⅓ cup tapioca flour
⅓ cup cornstarch
½ teaspoon xanthan gum

Cream together the cream cheese and butter. Add the flours, cornstarch, and xanthan gum and mix well with a fork or pastry cutter. The dough will form a ball.

Roll out the dough between sheets of plastic wrap dusted with rice flour. (It is easier to do this if you divide the dough into two or three sections.) Cut circles of pastry with a glass or a biscuit cutter and fit them into and up the sides of tartlet pans or small muffin tins. (You may prefer to work the dough into small balls and press with the fingers into and up the sides of the tins.) Chill.

FILLING

8 ounces fresh mushrooms
¼ cup fresh parsley
5 green onions
3 tablespoons butter or margarine
2 tablespoons vegetable oil
½ teaspoon salt
¾ teaspoon ground marjoram
6 tablespoons grated Cheddar cheese
6 tablespoons GF bread crumbs

Finely chop the mushrooms in the food processor. Remove them and mince the parsley. Remove the parsley and mince the green onions, using 2 to 3 inches of the green stem.

In a frying pan, heat the butter and oil. Add the minced vegetables and sauté over medium heat for about 6 minutes. The vegetables will start to give off their liquid and thicken a little. Transfer mixture to a bowl and add the salt, marjoram, grated cheese, and bread crumbs. Mix well.

Divide the filling among the chilled tart shells. Bake in preheated 350° oven for 20 to 25 minutes. Let cool for 5 minutes before unmolding. *Makes approximately 2½ dozen small tartlets or 18 larger ones.*

To freeze, cool first and then wrap carefully. Reheat in microwave or in a 375° oven for about 7 to 10 minutes. Serve hot.

Nutrients per tart: Calories 140, Fat 11 g, Carbohydrate 9 g, Cholesterol 25 mg, Sodium 180 mg, Fiber 0, Protein 2 g

QUICHE BITES: Instead of the mushroom filling, use half of the recipe for Crustless Seafood Quiche on page 275. The baking time is the same as for the mushroom tarts.

Swedish Meatballs 350°

I live in a Scandinavian neighborhood and here no party is complete unless the table boasts at least one serving dish of these tiny, tasty meatballs.

1½ pounds extra-lean ground beef
¾ cup GF cereal, crushed, or GF bread crumbs
2 small eggs
2 tablespoons chili sauce
1 tablespoon instant minced onion
1 teaspoon salt
⅛ teaspoon pepper
½ teaspoon GF curry powder

Put all ingredients in a mixing bowl and knead together with hands until well mixed. Form into 1-inch balls and brown in a Teflon-coated or lightly oiled frying pan, turning or rolling them to get all sides crusty. Then place in a 9″ × 13″ baking pan and bake in preheated 350° oven for about 25 minutes.

You can make these a day ahead and warm them up to serve in a chafing dish with picks for eating. *Makes 2 dozen meatballs.*

Nutrients per meatball: Calories 120, Fat 5 g, Carbohydrate 17 g, Cholesterol 120 mg, Sodium 740 mg, Fiber 5 g, Protein 5 g

Guacamole Dip

This spirited avocado dip is a natural for our diet, for it goes best with Fritos or corn tortilla chips.

2 ripe avocados
1 tablespoon grated onion
1 tablespoon lemon juice
1 teaspoon salt
¼ teaspoon chili powder
⅓ cup mayonnaise
Hot sauce or a salsa to taste

Peel the avocados and mash in a bowl with a fork. Stir in the onion, lemon juice, salt, and chili powder. Blend in the mayonnaise. Add the hot sauce or a salsa to taste, depending on how hot you like it. Cover tightly with plastic wrap and chill. Serve with corn or tortilla chips. *Makes approximately 1 cup of dip.*

Nutrients per tablespoon: Calories 35, Fat 3 g, Carbohydrate 2 g, Cholesterol 0, Sodium 300 mg, Fiber 1 g, Protein 0

Microwave Crab Dip

350°

For seafood lovers, a dip that spreads well on small rice crackers.

One 6-ounce can crab meat
One 3-ounce package cream cheese, softened
½ cup mayonnaise
¼ cup minced onion
1 tablespoon lemon juice
⅛ teaspoon Tabasco sauce

Drain and flake the crab meat. Beat the softened cream cheese until smooth. Stir in mayonnaise, crab meat, onion, lemon juice, and Tabasco sauce. Spoon into a small microwave dish. Microwave at Medium for 3 to

4 minutes, until bubbly. If you prefer, bake in a preheated 350° oven for 30 minutes. *Makes 1 cup of dip.*

Nutrients per tablespoon: Calories 160, Fat 16 g, Carbohydrate 1 g, Cholesterol 40 mg, Sodium 210 mg, Fiber 0, Protein 5 g

Granola

225°

I created this recipe originally as a gluten-free breakfast cereal for myself. I discovered it's great as a snack or in a survival packet on trips, and it is especially tasty made up into granola bars.

6 cups GF puffed rice
1 cup dry-roasted soybeans
1 cup unsweetened flake coconut
1 cup sunflower seeds (if unsalted, add ½ teaspoon salt)
¼ cup honey
¼ cup vegetable oil
2 cups raisins

Preheat oven to 225°. Grease a large roaster with vegetable oil spray. Put in the puffed rice, soybeans, coconut, and sunflower seeds.

In a saucepan, combine the honey and oil and heat to boiling. Watch and stir constantly because the mixture has a tendency to foam over the minute it comes to a boil. Remove from the heat and drizzle over the mixture in the roaster. Stir in well.

Bake at 225° for 2 hours, stirring every 30 minutes to keep the mixture from sticking together. Then add the raisins and turn off the oven. Put the pan back in the oven and let the granola cool down and dry out. (This can easily be left overnight.) Store airtight in cans. *Makes 10 cups granola, 20 servings.*

NOTE: This basic recipe can be varied as your taste dictates. Replace raisins with other dried fruit, coconut with chopped nuts. Add pine nuts with the sunflower seeds. Try popped corn, chopped in a food processor, instead of all puffed rice. Add grated orange rind. The variety is endless.

Nutrients per ½ cup serving: Calories 190, Fat 9 g, Carbohydrate 23 g, Cholesterol 0, Sodium 55 mg, Fiber 1 g, Protein 6 g

Granola Bars

350°

Marvelous for lunches, travel, hiking, or just plain snacking. The preceding recipe for granola makes enough for plenty of breakfast cereal plus these bars, or two batches of bars.

½ cup brown sugar
¼ cup dark corn syrup
⅓ cup sweetened condensed milk
2 tablespoons butter or margarine, melted
½ teaspoon vanilla
4½ cups Granola (page 263), chopped in a food processor to very coarse granules

Preheat oven to 350°. Grease a 9″ × 13″ oblong pan.

Mix the brown sugar, corn syrup, condensed milk, butter, and vanilla together well. Pour over the granola and mix thoroughly. It will be sticky.

Butter your hands and flatten the mixture into the prepared pan. Bake at 350° for 20 minutes.

Let cool about 10 minutes and cut into 1½ × 3-inch bars. If you wait longer, they will be hard to cut. *Makes 20 bars.*

Nutrients per bar: Calories 190, Fat 9 g, Carbohydrate 25 g, Cholesterol 5 mg, Sodium 25 mg, Fiber 3 g, Protein 4 g

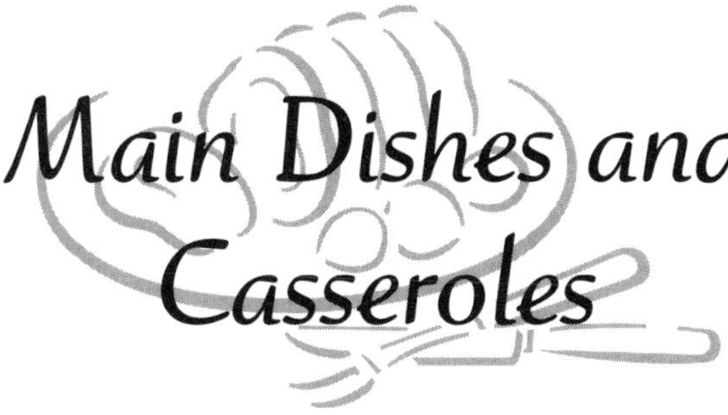

Main Dishes and Casseroles

Crowd Pleasers

Sauces for Casseroles

See Also

When I first started my gluten-free diet, I was content eating plain meats, potatoes, vegetables, and rice—and recovering my health. But it wasn't long before I found I craved the variety of flavors found only in mixed dishes, those bubbly with sauce, crunchy with varied textures, and rich with the odor of several foods combined.

In talking to other celiacs, I discovered that for most persons on a gluten-free diet, the steady fare of simply cooked meats and potatoes or rice becomes monotonous. Although we should remain suspicious and forgo that wonderful-smelling hot dish at a friend's table or at a restaurant, mixed dishes need not be forbidden at home.

In this section I include dishes that are favorites not only of mine but of my family and guests. As the cook, I don't like to prepare two separate meals; but I want others at the table to enjoy my GF food. Thus I've worked to make these mixed dishes both gluten free and tasty.

Many of these use rice, others potatoes, and some use nongluten bread. For the last, I use up my bread-making mistakes or buy a gluten-free rice bread sold in some health food stores or ordered by mail (see the section on gluten-free products at the end of the book).

Brown Rice Pilaf

A popular, easy-to-make, nutty-tasting rice dish to accompany barbecued ribs, baked chicken, or other meats that don't have drippings from which to make gravy. Serve it plain; the texture and flavor are so good it needs no sauce.

1 cup uncooked brown rice
2½ cups beef stock
2 teaspoons instant minced onion
1 teaspoon salt (if stock is unsalted)
1 tablespoon butter or margarine

Wash brown rice thoroughly and drain.

Bring stock, minced onion, and salt (if used) to a boil. Add rice and butter. Bring back to a boil and stir.

Lower heat until water is just bubbling. Cover and simmer 45 to 50 minutes. Turn off the heat. Remove lid and let stand 5 minutes to dry out.

To serve with chicken or turkey, I use chicken-flavored stock and add a stalk of celery thinly sliced. *Makes 3 cups of cooked rice, about 6 servings.*

Nutrients per serving: Calories 140, Fat 3 g, Carbohydrate 24 g, Cholesterol 5 mg, Sodium 400 mg, Fiber 2 g, Protein 4 g

PILAF PLUS: For a tasty variation of the basic recipe, add to the rice when you stir it into the stock ½ to 1 cup sliced raw mushrooms and ¼ to ½ cup grated raw carrots.

Sausage Rice Casserole 325°

A good way to use leftover pilaf, this moist meal-in-a-dish casserole is a favorite in our family. For a very easy meal, serve with tossed salad and fruit for dessert.

1 pound bulk pork or turkey sausage
2 cups cooked brown rice or Brown Rice Pilaf (page 268)
2 tablespoons diced onion
½ cup diced celery
One recipe Creamed Soup Base (cooked) (page 292)

In frying pan, brown the sausage. Drain off excess fat.

Place all ingredients in casserole and mix. Bake in preheated 325° oven for 50 to 60 minutes. *Makes 4 or 5 servings.*

Nutrients per serving: Calories 520, Fat 28 g, Carbohydrate 47 g, Cholesterol 65 mg, Sodium 205 mg, Fiber 3 g, Protein 18 g

Broccoli Rice Supreme 325°

This combination of vegetables, rice, and cheese is an all-around winner. For the cook it's easy to fix, can be done ahead, and freezes well, both before final cooking or as leftovers afterward. I think ½ to 1 cup diced ham is a nice addition to this dish, but it is delicious without it.

1 cup uncooked white rice
One 10-ounce box frozen chopped broccoli
½ cup minced onion
½ cup thinly sliced celery
2 tablespoons butter or margarine
½ to ¾ cup grated cheese
One 4-ounce can sliced mushrooms, drained
Double recipe Creamed Soup Base (cooked) (page 292), using the liquid from mushrooms as part of liquid

Cook rice in 2 cups of water, following recipe on box or bag. Cook broccoli and drain thoroughly. Sauté onion and celery in butter until onion is clear.

Line large greased casserole or 9″ × 13″ glass baking dish with rice. Mix the other ingredients together and pour over the rice. Refrigerate until ready to cook. This may be heated in the microwave approximately 6 to 8 minutes on high, until heated through, or baked in a preheated oven 45 minutes at 325°. *Makes 8 servings.*

If you add diced chicken or ham, you will have a full meal in a dish.

Nutrients per serving: Calories 180, Fat 7 g, Carbohydrate 25 g, Cholesterol 20 mg, Sodium 120 mg, Fiber 2 g, Protein 6 g

Chinese Fried Rice

This is the Chinese trick for stretching a little leftover meat (pork, chicken, or beef) into a whole main dish and is another tasty way of using leftover rice, either white or brown.

¼ to ½ cup cooked meat
2 tablespoons oil
2 green onions, thinly sliced
2 cups cooked brown or white rice
½ teaspoon salt
1 large egg
1½ tablespoons soy sauce
Minced parsley for garnish, if desired

Cut meat in thin slivers.

Heat oil in large skillet. Add green onions, and sauté about 2 minutes. Add meat and just heat through. Then add rice and salt and stir until all ingredients are blended. Beat egg with soy sauce and add to the rice, stirring rapidly so the mixture blends with the rice before setting. Cook until egg mixture is absorbed and the rice seems dry. This takes only a few minutes. Serve this Asian style by pressing rice into a bowl with a rounded bottom and then turning it out into a shallow dish, with the top now rounded. Garnish with minced parsley if you like. *Makes 4 servings.*

Nutrients per serving: Calories 220, Fat 10 g, Carbohydrate 23 g, Cholesterol 70 mg, Sodium 710 mg, Fiber 2 g, Protein 10 g

My Favorite Meat Loaf 350°

This is a firm meat loaf that tastes delicious either hot or cold. It slices well when cold and makes great sandwiches.

1 pound extra-lean ground beef
1 egg
1 teaspoon instant minced onion
1 tablespoon chili sauce
⅓ cup GF cereal, crushed (see Note)
Salt and pepper to taste

Place all ingredients in a mixing bowl and knead together with hands until well mixed. Form into a rounded shape and place in a flat pan that has low raised sides to contain any drippings. Bake in a preheated 350° oven for 50 to 60 minutes. Let stand for 5 minutes before cutting in thin slices. *Makes 4 servings.*

For a moister, more flavorful meatloaf, top it with this sauce: In a small bowl, mix ¼ cup ketchup, 2 teaspoons brown sugar, and ½ teaspoon prepared mustard. Spoon over loaf before baking.

NOTE: You may crush gluten-free rice or corn cereals, or save your bread mistakes or leftover bread and dry this in the oven. Then put in a blender or food processor and grind into crumbs. (Be sure to dry the bread first.)

Nutrients per serving: Calories 340, Fat 22 g, Carbohydrate 2 g, Cholesterol 150 mg, Sodium 130 mg, Fiber 0, Protein 30 g

Meatballs Pia

350°

This recipe for meatballs baked in a tasty sauce came from an Italian friend in Alaska. The combination of the American cranberry with an Italian-flavored meat sauce is unusual but good.

MEATBALLS

2 pounds ground meat
1 cup cornflakes
⅓ cup chopped parsley
2 eggs
2 tablespoons soy sauce
¼ teaspoon pepper
⅓ cup ketchup
2 tablespoons dry minced onion

SAUCE

One 12-ounce bottle chili sauce
1 tablespoon lemon juice
2 tablespoons brown sugar
One 16-ounce can cranberry jelly

In a bowl, mix together the meat, cornflakes, parsley, eggs, soy sauce, pepper, ketchup, and dry onion. Form into 1-inch meatballs. Brown slightly in a preheated 350° oven while you are mixing the sauce.

In a saucepan, place the chili sauce, lemon juice, brown sugar, and cranberry jelly. Heat until smooth and blended. Pour over the browned meatballs. Bake 30 to 35 minutes in 350° oven. *Makes 6 to 8 servings.*

Nutrients per serving: Calories 490, Fat 25 g, Carbohydrate 42 g, Cholesterol 120 mg, Sodium 1110 mg, Fiber 1 g, Protein 24 g

Monte Cristo Sandwich

A brunch or lunch favorite combining bread, meat, cheese, and eggs in one easy-to-serve hot sandwich. This recipe makes four sandwiches but could easily be cut to make a single portion.

8 slices GF bread
2 tablespoons mayonnaise
1 tablespoon mustard
4 thin slices cooked ham
4 slices Swiss cheese
4 slices turkey or chicken
Butter or margarine to spread
2 eggs
1 tablespoon milk or nondairy liquid

Lay out the 8 slices of bread. In a small bowl, combine the mayonnaise and mustard. Spread 4 slices of bread with the mixture. Top with 1 slice each of ham, cheese, and turkey. Spread butter on the other 4 bread slices and complete the sandwiches.

Whisk together the eggs and milk. Dip the sandwiches (both sides) in the egg-milk mixture and cook on a preheated oiled griddle over medium (or slightly lower) heat until browned. Turn and brown other side. Try to cook each side about 5 minutes so the sandwiches will be heated through.

Serve to be eaten with knife and fork. This goes well with the Hot Curried Fruit on page 177 for brunch or with potato chips for a luncheon.

Nutrients per serving: Calories 420, Fat 24 g, Carbohydrate 36 g, Cholesterol 175 mg, Sodium 590 mg, Fiber 4 g, Protein 17 g

No-Fail Cheese Soufflé   350°

An easy soufflé that doesn't fall when you serve it. This is a fine luncheon dish, but with its rich cheese flavor, it is also a good meatless dinner. I like it with a topping of heated Mushroom Soup made from the Creamed Soup Base (page 292).

1½ cups milk or nondairy liquid
2 cups soft GF bread crumbs
1½ cups grated Cheddar cheese
1 tablespoon butter
⅛ teaspoon paprika
1 teaspoon salt
3 eggs

In the top of a double boiler, place milk, bread crumbs, grated cheese, butter, and seasonings. Heat over hot water until the cheese is melted. Remove from heat and let cool slightly.

Meanwhile, separate the eggs. Beat the yolks slightly and add to the mixture in the double boiler. Beat whites until stiff. Fold them gently into the mixture. Pour into a greased 8″ × 8″ × 2″ baking dish set in a pan of hot water. Bake in a preheated 350° oven about 30 to 40 minutes, or until firm. Serve immediately. *Makes 6 servings.*

Any leftovers will keep in the refrigerator and can be reheated to serve at a later time.

Nutrients per serving: Calories 390, Fat 17 g, Carbohydrate 44 g, Cholesterol 150 mg, Sodium 450 mg, Fiber 2 g, Protein 16 g

Crustless Seafood Quiche

350°

Who says real men don't eat quiche? This is a favorite with the men who've tasted it. There is no need for a crust because the rice flour forms a rich brown skin on the bottom of the quiche. For the cook's convenience, the batter may be made as far as a day ahead and refrigerated.

½ cup sliced mushrooms
2 tablespoons butter or margarine
4 eggs
1 cup sour cream or nondairy substitute (low fat is fine)
1 cup small-curd cottage cheese (low fat is fine)
¼ cup sweet rice flour
¼ teaspoon salt
2 cups grated Monterey Jack cheese
6 ounces shrimp or crab meat

Sauté mushrooms in butter, then drain on a paper towel.

In a large mixing bowl, blend the eggs, sour cream, cottage cheese, rice flour, and salt. Stir in mushrooms, grated cheese, and shrimp. Pour into a 9″ or 10″ quiche dish or deep pie plate sprayed with Pam or greased lightly.

Bake 45 minutes in preheated 350° oven, or until knife inserted near center comes out clean. Let stand 5 minutes before cutting. *Makes 6 servings.*

Nutrients per serving: Calories 400, Fat 29 g, Carbohydrate 9 g, Cholesterol 235 mg, Sodium 511 mg, Fiber 0, Protein 25 g

HAM AND CHEESE QUICHE: Substitute ½ to ¾ cup diced ham for the shrimp or crab and use a small onion, diced, instead of the mushrooms.

Tamale Casserole 350°

This corn dish makes a good change from potatoes and rice. When I first served this casserole to my husband, he asked why I always experimented on him. I replied that it was because he is a meat-and-potatoes man. When he went back for a second helping larger than the first, I knew this was a success.

- **1 small onion, chopped**
- **½ medium green pepper, chopped**
- **1 clove garlic, minced**
- **1 tablespoon vegetable oil**
- **¾ pound lean ground beef**
- **One 8-ounce can tomato sauce**
- **One 8-ounce can whole-kernel corn**
- **One 6½-ounce can sliced black olives**
- **1 cup milk or nondairy liquid**
- **½ cup cornmeal**
- **½ teaspoon salt**
- **1 to 1½ teaspoons chili powder**
- **¾ cup grated sharp Cheddar cheese**

Sauté onion, pepper, and garlic in oil until onion is clear. Add beef and cook until browned. Pour off excess fat.

Add tomato sauce, drained corn, three-fourths of the olives, and the milk. Stir well, heat through, then add cornmeal, salt, and chili powder. Pour into well-greased 2-quart casserole. Decorate top with remaining olives.

Bake, covered, in preheated 350° oven for 45 minutes. Uncover and bake about 20 minutes more. For the last 5 minutes of baking, sprinkle cheese over the dish. It is ready when a knife inserted in center comes out clean. *Makes 4 or 5 servings.* Recipe can easily be doubled.

Nutrients per serving: Calories 600, Fat 26 g, Carbohydrate 63 g, Cholesterol 85 mg, Sodium 720 mg, Fiber 7 g, Protein 30 g

Mayonnaise Chicken Casserole

325°

A fine, moist casserole that can be made ahead and refrigerated before baking. This can be changed in many ways. Delete the mushrooms. Change the chicken to cooked ground turkey and add poultry seasoning to make it taste like turkey and dressing.

Butter or margarine
6 slices GF bread
2 cups cooked chicken
¼ cup diced onion
½ cup sliced celery
One 6½-ounce can sliced mushrooms, or ⅓ pound fresh mushrooms, sliced
¾ teaspoon salt
Dash of pepper
2 tablespoons sweet rice flour
2 eggs
½ cup mayonnaise
2½ cups milk or nondairy liquid

Butter bread and cut into cubes. Toss chicken, onion, celery, drained mushrooms, seasonings, and sweet rice flour together.

In a buttered 2-quart casserole, layer one-third of the bread with half the chicken mixture. Add one-third more bread and rest of mixture. Top with bread.

Beat the eggs slightly. Blend in mayonnaise and milk until smooth. Pour this over bread and chicken.

Bake in preheated 325° oven for 1 hour, until set. *Makes 4 servings.*

Nutrients per serving: Calories 640, Fat 45 g, Carbohydrate 31 g, Cholesterol 230 mg, Sodium 1080 mg, Fiber 3 g, Protein 32 g

Bette's Best Chicken Potpie 350°

After watching my husband order chicken potpie at restaurants, I realized I was denying him, as well as myself, this old favorite. When I tried one at home, it was so successful that he now compares all others to mine. The secret is the topping of tender buttermilk biscuits. With a tossed salad, this makes a complete meal.

1 cup cooked chicken
2 cups chicken stock
½ cup diced carrots
½ cup sliced celery
¼ cup minced onion
½ cup frozen peas
3 tablespoons rice flour
2 to 3 tablespoons water
¼ cup cream or nondairy substitute
Salt and pepper to taste
1 recipe Buttermilk Biscuit dough (page 83), sugar omitted

Dice the chicken and set aside. Place chicken stock in a large saucepan and bring to a boil. Add carrots, celery, and onions and cook for 15 minutes. Then add peas and chicken and cook 5 minutes longer.

Mix the rice flour to a thin paste with a few tablespoons of water. Thicken the stock with the rice flour paste and cook on low for a minute or two. Add cream and season with salt and pepper. (If the stock is salted, you probably won't need any more.)

Pour the cooked potpie mixture into a 2-quart casserole and top with 2½-inch rounds of biscuit dough. Bake all together in a preheated 350° oven for about 20 to 25 minutes. *Makes 5 or 6 servings.*

This recipe can be made ahead and refrigerated to be baked just before serving. The biscuits still rise but might take a bit longer to bake. Watch the oven and check the cooking. When the filling is bubbly and the biscuits a warm brown, the dish is ready to serve.

Nutrients per serving: Calories 150, Fat 5 g, Carbohydrate 15 g, Cholesterol 25 mg, Sodium 670 mg, Fiber 2 g, Protein 12 g

Easy Scalloped Potatoes 375°

Using the creamed soup base with a little butter or margarine makes creamy scalloped potatoes with little fuss and bother. Put the casserole in the oven and take time out to relax before dinner, or if you know you're going to be late, stir this up before work and have one of the kids put it in the oven when they get home from school.

5 fist-sized potatoes
5 to 7 green onions, thinly sliced
Salt and pepper to taste
½ cup leftover or deli ham or corned beef, diced (optional)

SAUCE
2 tablespoons butter or margarine
4 tablespoons Creamed Soup Base (page 292)
¼ cup cold water
1¼ cups chicken stock
1 cup milk or nondairy substitute

Preheat oven to 375°. Grease a 2½-quart casserole with cooking spray.

Peel and thinly slice the potatoes into the casserole. Stir in the onions and ham (if using). Add salt and pepper to taste.

Sauce: In a medium saucepan, place the butter and soup base blended with the cold water. Add the chicken stock and bring to a boil over medium-high heat, stirring occasionally. This will be as thick as canned cream soup. Add the milk and pour over the potatoes. Bake for 1 hour, or until the potatoes are tender. *Makes 4 or 5 servings.*

Nutrients per serving (without ham): Calories 230, Fat 4 g, Carbohydrate 37 g, Cholesterol 25 mg, Sodium 440 mg, Fiber 1 g, Protein 11 g

POTATOES AU GRATIN: Eliminate the meat and add 1 cup grated sharp Cheddar cheese to the sauce before pouring it onto the potatoes. If desired, top with ½ cup buttered GF bread crumbs.

VARIATION: If you prefer the mushroom taste to green onion, try using the recipe for Mushroom Soup (page 292) and thinning it with the cup of milk before pouring over the potatoes.

Gone-for-the-Day Stew

225°

This easy but delicious stew was created by one of my skiing friends who didn't want to steal from her time on the slopes to cook. She stuck the casserole in the oven after breakfast, and we'd return tired and hungry at the end of the day to a full main dish ready and waiting.

1 to 1½ pounds beef stew meat
One 24-ounce package frozen stew vegetables (see Note)
One recipe Creamed Soup Base or Cream of Chicken Soup (page 292)
One 13-ounce can onion soup
One 14½-ounce can beef broth

Brown the meat. Place in a 4-quart casserole or dutch oven, then toss in all the other ingredients. Cover. Put dish in an oven set at 225° and forget it for 6 to 8 hours. Serve. There is no extra work here, for the combination of soups makes a zesty, creamy gravy seasoned to perfection. This also makes a good overnight Crock-Pot dish. *Makes 6 to 8 servings.*

NOTE: Or use ½ cup small pearl onions, 1 cup celery cut in ⅓-inch slices, 1½ cups carrots sliced in ½-inch slices, and 1½ cups small round potatoes or larger potatoes cut into 1- to 1½-inch chunks.

Nutrients per serving: Calories 490, Fat 9 g, Carbohydrate 49 g, Cholesterol 30 mg, Sodium 510 mg, Fiber 2 g, Protein 25 g

Sausage and Lentil Bake

The high protein in lentils plus the spicy sausage make this a winner for taste and nutrition. This makes a large dish and is even better the next day, or frozen and heated again for another meal.

1 cup dried lentils
2 cups water
2 teaspoons instant beef broth granules
8 ounces kielbasa sausage
One 16-ounce can tomatoes
1 cup sliced celery
1 cup chopped onions
1 teaspoon dried minced garlic
¼ cup ketchup
1 teaspoon prepared mustard
3 tablespoons brown sugar

Wash lentils and pick over carefully. Drain. Put water and broth granules in 4-quart dutch oven and bring to boil over high heat. Meanwhile, cut sausage into ¼-inch-thick rounds. Purée the tomatoes. Prepare other vegetables.

Add all the ingredients to the stock and let contents come back to boil. Boil briskly for about 30 seconds, stirring constantly.

Reduce heat to low. Cover the pot, leaving lid slightly ajar. Simmer 45 to 50 minutes, until lentils are tender. If mixture seems too thick, stir in ¼ cup water. Serve with a tossed salad for a full meal. *Makes 6 to 8 servings.*

Nutrients per serving: Calories 180, Fat 4 g, Carbohydrate 26 g, Cholesterol 15 mg, Sodium 510 mg, Fiber 3 g, Protein 10 g

Easy Enchiladas
350°

Don't pass this one up! I served it to unexpected company, and they raved. It takes only a few minutes to prepare and about 15 minutes to cook.

1 pound ground beef
One 8-ounce can tomato sauce
1 package enchilada sauce mix
1½ cups water
8 thick corn tortillas
½ cup grated Cheddar cheese

In a frying pan, brown the ground beef. Meanwhile, combine tomato sauce, enchilada sauce mix, and water in saucepan. Bring to a boil; simmer 5 minutes.

Drain fat off the ground beef and stir ½ cup of sauce into meat.

Dip each tortilla into sauce. Put 3 tablespoons meat filling on each. Roll tortillas around filling and place, seam sides down, in 8″ × 12″ × 2″ baking dish.

Spread remaining sauce evenly over enchiladas and top with grated cheese. Bake in a preheated 350° oven for 15 minutes, or slightly longer if desired. *Makes 4 servings.*

Nutrients per serving: Calories 530, Fat 27 g, Carbohydrate 35 g, Cholesterol 115 mg, Sodium 1080 mg, Fiber 1 g, Protein 35 g

Crowd Pleasers

For celiacs, going past the hot dishes at a picnic or potluck supper is as frustrating as walking past a bakery. We have to avoid every mixed dish, for many obviously contain pasta. Other dishes are suspect, for they might contain gluten in the form of canned creamed soups or wheat-flour thickening.

To avoid this disappointment, take your own main dish. The following have proved popular with my guests, and are safely gluten free.

Homemade Chili

Chili is a simple crowd pleaser, especially a young crowd. It's easy to make, inexpensive, and gluten free.

2 pounds ground beef
1 large onion, chopped, plus 3 tablespoons finely chopped onion, for garnish
Two 28-ounce cans stewed tomatoes
Two 15-ounce cans chili beans
One 15-ounce can kidney beans
One or two 6-ounce cans Spicy Hot V8 vegetable juice
2 tablespoons sugar
2 tablespoons chili powder
½ teaspoon garlic powder
¾ teaspoon onion powder
½ cup grated Cheddar cheese, for garnish

Brown meat in a large kettle. Add chopped onion and cook until onion is clear. Add remaining ingredients except garnishes, using the bean liquid and as much of the Spicy Hot V8 as you need to achieve the desired consistency. Simmer on back of stove for at least 1 hour, preferably longer. For an added touch, serve topped with grated Cheddar cheese and finely chopped raw onion. *Makes 18 to 20 servings.*

This may be made a day ahead and reheated, or may simmer for hours on the stove until ready to serve.

Nutrients per serving: Calories 280, Fat 14 g, Carbohydrate 21 g, Cholesterol 60 mg, Sodium 770 mg, Fiber 4 g, Protein 19 g

Calico Beans 350°

This mixture of several kinds of beans with the ground beef gives it a different flavor from the usual baked bean hot dishes at potlucks and picnics. This recipe makes a lot and can be mixed up ahead of time and baked at the last hour. Any leftovers can be frozen, but because this is a favorite with men and boys, there are seldom any leftovers.

4 or 5 strips bacon
1 pound extra-lean ground beef
One 28-ounce can GF pork and beans
One 15-ounce can kidney beans
One 17-ounce can small lima beans
½ cup ketchup
1 teaspoon salt
¾ cup brown sugar
1 teaspoon prepared mustard
2 tablespoons wine vinegar

Cut bacon into small bits. Brown it in a skillet with the beef. Drain off any extra fat. Put in a large casserole and add beans, drained slightly.

Mix ketchup, salt, brown sugar, mustard, and vinegar and stir into the beans and meat mixture. This can now be refrigerated until 40 minutes before serving time or baked and then reheated for serving.

Bake 40 minutes in a preheated 350° oven. *Makes 18 to 20 servings.*

Nutrients per serving: Calories 180, Fat 6 g, Carbohydrate 24 g, Cholesterol 20 mg, Sodium 490 mg, Fiber 5 g, Protein 10 g

Hawaiian Curry

Before I was served this marvelous mild, sweet curry in Hawaii, I was sure I could never learn to enjoy this unusual dish. But it is not at all like the strong Indian curries. I have served it often to others who aren't fond of curry and have always had compliments.

It takes more time to prepare than the other dishes for a crowd, so save this for your favorite guests. They will love you for it.

1 medium onion
2 cloves garlic
3 inches fresh gingerroot
¾ cup (1½ sticks) butter or margarine
¾ cup sweet rice flour
¼ cup curry powder (see Notes)
Salt to taste
¼ cup sugar
2 cups chicken broth
2 cups milk or nondairy liquid
One 7¾-ounce can coconut milk (see Notes)
3 cups cubed cooked chicken

Chop the onion, mince the garlic, and grate the gingerroot. Sauté these in the butter in a large pan. Add the flour, curry, salt, and sugar. Do not allow mixture to burn or lump. Slowly add the chicken broth and cook until well blended and smooth. Boil a little, stirring constantly.

Add milk and coconut milk; do not let boil. Add the cubed chicken and put pan over hot water. Keep water at a simmer and cook the curry for 4 hours, stirring often. You may need to add more chicken broth if sauce gets too thick, or more sugar or salt to taste. *Makes 12 to 16 servings.*

Serve your curry with cooked white rice and an assortment of the traditional condiments: mango chutney, bacon bits, chopped macadamia nuts, chopped green onion tops, shredded fresh coconut. Some people use chopped hard-boiled eggs, but I prefer to stuff the eggs and serve separately. I also like to serve Baked Bananas (page 176) as a side dish for this company spread.

This should serve 16, but most people come back for seconds and thirds, so plan on that. I double the recipe, going a bit easy on the flour. The amount of chicken can vary. It doesn't have to be doubled.

This is a good way to use your Thanksgiving or Christmas turkey leftovers to serve a crowd.

Nutrients per serving: Calories 430, Fat 29 g, Carbohydrate 13 g, Cholesterol 85 mg, Sodium 200 mg, Fiber 1 g, Protein 30 g

NOTES: Curry powder is a mixed spice, so check the ingredients list on the label.

If you can't find coconut milk, use shredded, unsweetened coconut to taste (about ¼ cup) and increase amount of milk by 1 cup.

Party Fruit Tray

This not only looks appetizing but can serve as either salad or dessert. And for many who dislike mixed fruit salads, this way of offering fruit in large serving-size pieces makes it more appealing.

NOTE: If taking this to a potluck or party at another site, always prepare the fruit (except the bananas) ahead of time and place the pieces in separate plastic bags to arrange on the tray at the party in order not to take up room in the hostess's kitchen.

1 head lettuce
1 fresh pineapple
1 ripe papaya
2 or 3 oranges
1 cantaloupe
2 or 3 bananas
1 pound red seedless grapes
3 kiwis
2 carambolas (star fruit)
2 tablespoons lemon juice

Wash the lettuce and line the tray, leaving the edges hanging over for decoration.

Prepare the large fruits by peeling and coring or seeding and cutting into large serving slices or wedges. Peel the oranges and slice. Cut the bananas into thirds on an angle. Peel and slice the kiwis. Wash and slice the carambolas.

Arrange on the tray in heaping sections of each fruit arranged around the grapes in the center. Sprinkle the bananas and papaya liberally with the lemon juice.

Cover with plastic wrap and keep in a cool place or refrigerator until serving. *Serves 12 to 16.*

Sauces for Casseroles

For the gluten-free cook there is no reaching for a can of cream soup to make an easy sauce since most of them contain wheat flour and have to be avoided. But with the handy Creamed Soup Base (page 292), you can have the equivalent in just minutes.

If you haven't made up the soup base yet, here are a couple of easy sauces for your casserole.

Cheese Sauce

This sauce goes well with casseroles using potatoes, rice, or pasta.

2 tablespoons chopped onion
1 tablespoon butter or margarine
1 tablespoon sweet rice flour
¾ cup chicken stock
2 cups milk or nondairy liquid
¾ cup grated Cheddar cheese
Salt and paprika for seasoning

In a saucepan, sauté the onion in the butter until clear. Then stir in the rice flour. Blend well.

Add the stock slowly, stirring as you pour it in. When the sauce is smooth and boiling, add the milk. Heat the soup but don't let it boil, and then add the grated cheese.

Season to taste with salt and paprika. Remember that if the stock is salted, you will probably need little additional salt. *Makes 3 cups of sauce.*

Nutrients per serving: Calories 270, Fat 19 g, Carbohydrate 11 g, Cholesterol 60 mg, Sodium 668 mg, Fiber 11 g, Protein 16 g

Mushroom Sauce

Here is a tasty, easy-to-make sauce for casseroles.

One 4-ounce can mushrooms, drained, or ½ cup sliced fresh mushrooms
1½ teaspoons dry minced onion
2 tablespoons rice flour
One 14-ounce can chicken stock
½ cup rich cream or nondairy liquid
Salt and pepper to taste

Place the mushrooms, minced onion, and rice flour in blender. Add ½ cup of the chicken stock. Blend slightly. Add the rest of the stock and blend again. The mushrooms can remain in small chunks or be minced.

Place the blended mix in a saucepan and cook until thickened. Then add the cream and cook a minute or two, stirring constantly. The sauce will be quite thick. At this point, season to taste. If the stock was salted, it will need very little more seasoning.

For use, thin to desired consistency with milk or nondairy liquid or with water for the casserole of your choice. *Makes about 3 cups of thick sauce.*

Nutrients per serving: Calories 160, Fat 6 g, Carbohydrate 26 g, Cholesterol 15 mg, Sodium 630 mg, Fiber 3 g, Protein 3 g

Soups and Chowders

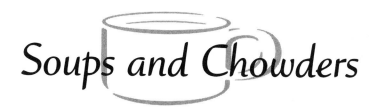

Soups Featuring Vegetables

Soups with Clams or Chicken

Soups Containing Beans, Peas, or Lentils

The day I was diagnosed and heard I would have to avoid gluten, I raced from the doctor's office to the store to find something quick to fix. I assumed soups would be safe. To my surprise, almost every can contained wheat flour or modified food starch. In desperation I grabbed a can of vegetable soup without the word *starch* or *wheat* on the label and hurried home to open it.

When I poured it into the pan, I saw, mixed in with the vegetable chunks, little round spots of barley—another of the forbidden gluten grains. I dumped the soup down the garbage disposal unit.

You've probably discovered, as I did, that most canned soups contain one of these three: barley, gluten for thickening, or pasta for body. And your hunger for soup is probably as keen as mine was when I poured out that vegetable soup and settled for peanut butter on a rice cake.

Soups in a restaurant can also be poison for a celiac. Chowders and cream soups are invariably thickened with wheat flour, while poultry and vegetable soups will contain either noodles or barley, or both. Even powdered and dried soups must be suspect. They often contain wheat starch for thickening, although there are some that are gluten free. Some are available by mail (see pages 309–15), and a few can be found on the grocery shelves.

Probably the most exciting discovery in the last ten years is finding a great substitute for that can of creamed soup for a casserole. See the easy Creamed Soup Base at the beginning of the chapter. No GF home should be without this mix.

Creamed Soup Base

The days of opening that handy can of thick condensed creamed soup for the casserole or hot dish is over for the wheat intolerant, but if you keep this dry powdered base right by your kitchen stove, you can make the equivalent of that can of thick chicken, mushroom, or other creamed soup in about 3 minutes—almost as fast as opening a can. And it takes up only the room of a pint jar. Use it also as a cream sauce or thin it for chicken gravy.

NOTE: For vegetarians there are some vegetable soup bases on the market. For the lactose intolerant, use the powdered baby formula Isomil (soy) or Pregestimil (corn) instead of Lacto-Free nondairy dry powder for the best flavor.

1 cup dry milk powder or nondairy substitute (see Note above)
1 cup white rice flour
2 tablespoons dried minced onions
½ teaspoon pepper
½ teaspoon salt
3 tablespoons GF powdered soup base (chicken or vegetable)

Combine all ingredients and mix well. Store in an airtight container by your kitchen stove or on the pantry shelf. *This mix is the equivalent of 8 or 9 cans of soup.*

CREAM OF CHICKEN SOUP: In a small saucepan, blend 4 tablespoons of base with ¼ cup cold water. Add 1 cup hot water (or chicken stock) and cook over medium heat, stirring until the soup thickens.

CREAM OF MUSHROOM SOUP: Follow the instructions for Cream of Chicken Soup using the liquid from one 4-ounce can of mushroom bits and pieces as part of the water (reserving the mushrooms). After the soup thickens, add the mushrooms.

CREAM OF TOMATO SOUP: Follow the instructions for Cream of Chicken Soup, using one 5.5-ounce can of V8 juice as part of the liquid.

CHEESE SOUP OR SAUCE: Follow the instructions for Cream of Chicken Soup, using ¼ cup of the base. Add ¼ cup extra water. Stir in ½ to ⅔ cup grated Cheddar cheese before removing from the stove.

SHRIMP SOUP OR SAUCE: Follow the instructions for Cream of Chicken Soup. Use one 8-ounce bottle clam juice plus the ¼ cup water and add one 4½-ounce can broken shrimp (drained) or ½ cup cut-up cooked shrimp before removing from the stove.

TASTY CREAM SAUCE: Melt 1 tablespoon butter or margarine in a small saucepan and add 1 teaspoon chopped chives or 2 thinly sliced green onions before putting in the soup base. Add 1¼ cups hot water and cook as directed for Cream of Chicken Soup.

TO USE IN A CASSEROLE: If your casserole (scalloped potatoes, etc.) calls for canned soup and is to be baked more than 1 hour, just stir the Creamed Soup Base with the ingredients and pour on 1¼ to 1½ cups hot water.

Soups Featuring Vegetables

Quick Vegetable Soup

If you're lucky enough to have a small pressure cooker, this soup can be made in minutes and tastes like the old-fashioned, long-simmered soup of yesterday.

If you don't, this soup can be simmered slowly with the same results. Using beef stock instead of some of the water will help the flavor, but remember to reduce the salt if the stock is salted.

¼ pound lean ground beef
3 cups hot water
½ cup diced carrots
¼ cup diced onion
½ cup sliced celery
One 8-ounce can V8 juice
½ cup chopped cabbage
1 tablespoon chopped parsley
1 teaspoon salt
⅛ teaspoon pepper

Brown the beef in the pressure cooker. Add the rest of the ingredients. Cover, set control at 15, and cook for 3 minutes after control jiggles. Remove from heat and let stand 5 minutes. Then reduce pressure by letting cold water run over the pan. *Makes 4 servings.*

Nutrients per serving: Calories 120, Fat 6 g, Carbohydrate 10 g, Cholesterol 20 mg, Sodium 820 mg, Fiber 2 g, Protein 6 g

Savory Minestrone

Almost all the canned minestrone soups include pasta as one ingredient and thus forbidden to a celiac. You can make the following soup without pasta or add GF pasta either purchased or made from the recipe on page 230.

This is an excellent full-meal soup. The combination of sweet sausage, vegetables, and beans fills most of your nutritional requirements. It is so good the whole family will enjoy it.

1 pound Italian sweet sausage
1 tablespoon vegetable oil
1 cup diced onion
1 clove garlic, minced
1 cup diced carrots
1 teaspoon crumbled basil
2 small zucchini, sliced
One 16-ounce can tomatoes, undrained
Two 14½-ounce cans beef stock (see Note)
2 cups shredded cabbage
1 teaspoon salt
¼ teaspoon pepper
One 16-ounce can Great Northern beans, undrained
¼ cup GF pasta (optional)

Slice sausage crosswise into ½-inch slices and brown in oil in a deep saucepan or Dutch oven. Add onion, garlic, carrots, and basil. Cook for 5 minutes. Add zucchini, tomatoes with their juice, beef stock, cabbage, salt, and pepper. Bring soup to a boil. Reduce heat and simmer, covered, for 1 hour. Add beans with their liquid and cook another 20 minutes. Add pasta if desired. This soup keeps well and tastes even better the next day. It also freezes well. *Makes 8 servings.*

NOTE: You may make the beef stock from gluten-free powdered beef bouillon. Follow the directions for 3½ cups stock.

Nutrients per serving: Calories 330, Fat 20 g, Carbohydrate 23 g, Cholesterol 55 mg, Sodium 1260 mg, Fiber 2 g, Protein 14 g

Daisy's Homemade Tomato Soup

Tomato soup from the market shelves usually contains some form of gluten, so during one summer of an abundant tomato harvest, I pulled out my mother's recipe for homemade tomato soup. This family recipe is easy to make and far better tasting than the canned soups.

I make this by the quart during tomato season when vine-ripened tomatoes are inexpensive and plentiful. Then I freeze the soup in 1-cup or 2-cup freezer containers for use all winter. It can be eaten as a soup after thawing and heating with the addition of cream or a nondairy substitute, or it can be used in many recipes calling for tomatoes or tomato soup.

1 quart ripe tomatoes, quartered
1 tablespoon sugar
¼ teaspoon salt
1 tablespoon dried minced onion
⅛ teaspoon tarragon

Wash tomatoes and cut up into saucepan. Mash slightly so there is juice in the bottom of the pan. Add the sugar, salt, onion, and tarragon and bring to a boil on medium or medium-low heat. Be sure to stir so the tomatoes don't stick to the bottom of the pan. After they reach a boil, turn down heat and simmer until tomatoes are soft. I like to leave them at least an hour for all the seasonings to blend together.

Put mixture through a Foley food mill to eliminate the skins and most of the seeds. Let the soup cool before filling your freezer cartons. To serve, thaw, heat, and add a dash of cream or nondairy substitute. Don't heat after the cream is added, as it tends to curdle.

If you don't have a food mill, peel the tomatoes before cooking, then purée the cooked soup in a blender or food processor.

I usually make this in 2-quart batches to save time. Just double all ingredients. The double batch will make 6 cups of soup plus enough for a taste for yourself. *Serving size: 1 cup.*

Nutrients per serving: Calories 35, Fat 0.5 g, Carbohydrate 8 g, Cholesterol 0, Sodium 95 mg, Fiber 2 g, Protein 1 g

Tomato Cheese Soup

In this soup the cheese is not cooked with the soup; it is put in the bowl and the broth poured over it, causing the cheese to turn to strings that trail from the spoon like the watches in a Dali painting.

2 teaspoons margarine or butter
1 tablespoon chopped onion
1 small clove garlic, minced
1 teaspoon chopped fresh cilantro (coriander)
1½ cups chicken broth (see Note)
1 tomato, peeled and chopped
Salt and pepper to taste
½ cup shredded Monterey Jack cheese
½ cup shredded Cheddar cheese

In a small saucepan, melt the margarine over medium heat; add onion and garlic and stir often until onion is clear. Stir in cilantro, broth, and tomato. Bring to a boil, cover, reduce heat, and simmer for about 10 minutes to blend flavors. Season to taste. (If broth is salted, you may not need more salt.)

Place equal portions of the cheeses in 2 large soup bowls. Ladle soup over cheese. *Makes 2 servings.*

This can easily be doubled or redoubled to serve 4 or 8.

NOTE: You may make your own stock from chicken backs and necks, use canned chicken broth, or use a powdered GF chicken soup base. For the latter, use 1 teaspoon (or less) of base per cup of water.

Nutrients per serving: Calories 310, Fat 22 g, Carbohydrate 8 g, Cholesterol 65 mg, Sodium 1930 mg, Fiber 1 g, Protein 21 g

Czechoslovakian Cabbage Soup

When my garage mechanic learned I was writing a cookbook, he gave me this favorite family recipe that he cooks up on his days off. After I tasted it, I begged permission to add it to the cookbook. This is not a quick-cooking soup, but one that tastes better for slow simmering—and even better heated up the next day.

This is a traditional country soup of Czechoslovakia. The beef bones, short ribs, vegetables, and seasonings make it hearty enough for a whole meal.

2 pounds beef soup bones
1 cup chopped onion
3 carrots, diced
2 cloves garlic, chopped
1 bay leaf
2 pounds beef short ribs
1 teaspoon dried thyme
1 teaspoon paprika
8 cups water
1 head cabbage, chopped (8 cups)
Two 16-ounce cans tomatoes, undrained
2 teaspoons salt
½ teaspoon Tabasco sauce
½ cup chopped parsley
3 tablespoons lemon juice
3 tablespoons sugar
One 16-ounce can sauerkraut, drained

Place beef bones, onion, carrots, garlic, and bay leaf in a roasting pan. Top with short ribs and sprinkle with thyme and paprika. Roast uncovered in preheated 450° oven for 20 minutes, until meat is browned.

Transfer meat and vegetables to a large kettle. Add water, cabbage, tomatoes and their liquid, salt, and Tabasco. Bring to a boil. Cover and simmer 1½ hours. Skim off fat.

Add parsley, lemon juice, sugar, and sauerkraut. Cook, uncovered, for 1 hour. Remove bones and short ribs from kettle. Trim meat from bones, cut into cubes, and return to the soup. Cook 5 minutes longer.

This will make 12 servings, but none ever goes to waste since it freezes well.

Nutrients per serving: Calories 540, Fat 28 g, Carbohydrate 11 g, Cholesterol 55 mg, Sodium 840 mg, Fiber 2 g, Protein 12 g

Pumpkin Soup

The special flavor in this soup comes from peanut butter. It sounds weird but tastes delicious. This recipe serves two, but it can be doubled or redoubled to serve a crowd.

1 tablespoon unsalted butter
1 cup pumpkin pie filling
½ cup puréed cooked sweet potatoes
¼ cup peanut butter
1½ cups chicken or turkey broth
¼ teaspoon pepper
¼ teaspoon salt (optional)

Melt butter in a saucepan over medium heat. Stir in pumpkin, sweet potatoes, and peanut butter.

Add broth, pepper, and salt if desired (you may not need salt if the broth is salted). Reduce heat and simmer 20 minutes.

Serve garnished, if you like, with a dab of sour cream or nondairy substitute sprinkled with chopped chives. *Makes 2 servings.*

Nutrients per serving: Calories 490, Fat 20 g, Carbohydrate 64 g, Cholesterol 10 mg, Sodium 1910 mg, Fiber 5 g, Protein 19 g

Potato Leek Soup

A hearty soup that reminds one of a cozy kitchen on a cold winter evening. Serve with warm bread, muffins, or biscuits for a full meal.

3 fist-sized potatoes
3 leeks
1 stalk celery
1 large carrot
¼ cup (½ stick) butter or margarine
¾ teaspoon salt
½ cup water
3 cups milk or nondairy liquid
Snippets of thyme, marjoram, and basil

Peel and cube the potatoes, clean and chop the leeks, chop the celery, and peel and dice the carrot. Place the prepared vegetables and the butter in a saucepan. Add the salt and cook over medium heat, stirring constantly, until butter is melted and the vegetables are coated.

Add the water and bring to a boil, then cover and simmer. Cook until the potatoes are tender, adding more water if needed.

Remove vegetables and purée with the milk in a food processor or blender. Return to saucepan and add herbs. Reheat but do not boil. *Makes 6½ cups, 6 servings.*

NOTE: If green stalks of the leeks are used, the soup will be green; if only the white part, the soup will be creamy white. It's good either way.

Nutrients per serving: Calories 250, Fat 12 g, Carbohydrate 29 g, Cholesterol 35 mg, Sodium 430 mg, Fiber 5 g, Protein 8 g

Microwave Potato Soup

I think of potato soup as a hearty cold-weather dish. This is quick and easy for the working man or woman to fix.

1 slice bacon, diced
1 medium-sized potato
⅛ teaspoon dried thyme
1 cup chicken broth
1 cup milk or nondairy liquid
Dash of pepper

Place bacon in a 1- to 1½-quart glass bowl. Cover and microwave on High until bacon is brown, 1 to 1½ minutes. Lift out bacon and drain on a paper towel.

Discard half the drippings. Peel and dice the potato and add with thyme to the remaining drippings. Cook on High until potato is tender, 4 to 6 minutes.

Mash the potato with a fork. Stir in broth and milk. Cover and cook on High, stirring once or twice, until steaming, 4 to 5 minutes. Season with pepper to taste and sprinkle with the bacon. *Makes 2 servings.*

Nutrients per serving: Calories 190, Fat 7 g, Carbohydrate 19 g, Cholesterol 20 mg, Sodium 910 mg, Fiber 4 g, Protein 13 g

Soups with Clams or Chicken

New England Clam Chowder

Canned clam chowders are usually thickened with wheat starch. There is no need for this because the potatoes in the chowder provide enough thickening. This recipe is quick to fix and filling enough for a main dish at lunch or supper.

1 medium onion
2 slices bacon
1 cup peeled and diced raw potatoes
One 6½-ounce can chopped clams
2 cups chicken stock
1 cup nondairy creamer or evaporated milk
1 cup water
Pepper to taste
½ teaspoon salt
3 or 4 tablespoons grated carrot for garnish (optional)

Chop the onion; mince the bacon. Fry the bacon gently until cooked but not crisp. Add onion and sauté until clear.

Meanwhile, dice the potatoes. Drain the clams, reserving the juice. Transfer the bacon and onion to a soup pan and add the potatoes, clam juice, and chicken stock. Cook until potatoes are tender.

Place half the mixture in a blender and blend until smooth. Return blended mixture to saucepan and add clams, nondairy liquid or evaporated milk, water, pepper, and salt. (If the chicken stock is salted, you may not need salt.) Heat and serve. If desired, just before serving add the grated carrot and cook a minute or two. The carrot adds color and texture to the soup. *Makes 1½ quarts, 6 to 8 servings.*

NOTE: You may leave the potatoes diced instead of blending them. In this case, thicken the soup with a thin paste of potato starch and water. Start with 2 tablespoons and let cook before adding more because the potato starch thickens about twice as much liquid as wheat flour paste. I cannot give an exact amount of starch, since potatoes have different thickening properties and people prefer different consistencies of chowder.

Nutrients per serving: Calories 100, Fat 4 g, Carbohydrate 12 g, Cholesterol 25 mg, Sodium 360 mg, Fiber 1 g, Protein 5 g

CLAM CORN CHOWDER: Add one 8-ounce can creamed corn to the clam chowder recipe before the chowder is thickened (the corn may change the consistency). The chowder may not need thickening. Be sure the corn is gluten free.

Chinese Corn Soup

This is a quick corn and chicken soup that makes a full meal. I clipped it from the newspaper and assumed it was an Americanized version of a Chinese dish until I was served this in China and discovered that my soup tasted exactly like that served in the Chinese restaurant in Canton.

This recipe can be found in Enjoy Chinese Cuisine *by Judy Lew, to whom the recipe was credited in the* Seattle Times.

2 whole chicken breasts, boned and skinned
1 egg white
1 tablespoon rice wine
1 tablespoon cornstarch
1 quart chicken stock
One 8-ounce can creamed corn
1 teaspoon salt
1½ teaspoons pepper
1 egg, beaten
2 tablespoons cornstarch dissolved in 2 tablespoons water

Dice the chicken breasts into bite-sized pieces or slice to thin slivers and combine with the egg white, rice wine, and cornstarch. Set aside.

Bring to a boil the chicken stock, creamed corn, salt, and pepper. (If the chicken stock is already salted, you will need to reduce the salt here. I use none until it is ready for the table and then salt to taste.) When stock reaches a boil, add the chicken pieces, stirring constantly to break up the chicken. Cook 1 minute.

Add the beaten egg in a thin stream, stirring slowly in one direction.

Thicken the soup with the cornstarch and water mixture, stirring for a few minutes. *Makes 6 to 8 servings,* depending on whether you use as a full meal or a soup course.

Nutrients per serving: Calories 160, Fat 4 g, Carbohydrate 9 g, Cholesterol 65 mg, Sodium 1180 mg, Fiber 1 g, Protein 21 g

Hearty Chicken Noodle Soup

The noodles used in canned soups contain gluten, so if you like noodles, you will have to make your own soups and add the GF products. You may use pure rice noodles or bean threads found in the Asian section of grocery stores, make your own from the pasta recipe on page 230, or order from one of the many suppliers (pages 309–15).

This hearty soup is a full meal at lunch and is excellent for the luncheon thermos, and even better if the worker has access to a microwave.

3 cups chicken stock
½ cup chopped celery
⅔ cup diced leftover cooked chicken or one 4- or 6-ounce can chicken
½ cup diced carrots
½ cup uncooked noodles
2 tablespoons butter or margarine
2 tablespoons rice flour
Salt to taste
1 tablespoon parsley flakes
½ cup cream or nondairy substitute (optional)

Simmer chicken stock, celery, chicken, and carrots until vegetables are tender, about 20 minutes. Add noodles and cook until they are done. (Bean threads take only a minute or two; rice noodles and homemade ones must be tested for doneness.)

Melt butter and mix with the flour, adding a small amount of the hot chicken stock. Stir this mixture into the simmering soup. Add salt and parsley flakes.

Heat the cream if using and add to the soup. The cream lightens the color of the soup. Let cook for a short while. Do not boil after adding the cream. *Makes 5 or 6 servings.*

Nutrients per serving: Calories 1130, Fat 8 g, Carbohydrate 250 g, Cholesterol 25 mg, Sodium 560 mg, Fiber 1 g, Protein 12 g

Soups Containing Beans, Peas, or Lentils

Bean, pea, and lentil soups do not need thickeners, but surprisingly a large number of commercial canners have added wheat flour to their products, thus forcing us to read labels carefully or to make our own soups.

They require little work but a long time on the stove, and all the recipes I've found make a large batch. If you can keep the rest of the family from taking too many second helpings, you will have enough left from the next three recipes to freeze for later use.

Split Pea Soup

This soup is so thick and hearty that it makes a full meal. And since split peas are high in fiber, its food value is as great as the soup tastes.

1 ham hock
7½ cups water
2½ cups dried split peas
1 cup chopped onion
2 cloves garlic, minced
1 carrot, diced
1 teaspoon salt (or to taste)
½ teaspoon pepper

Cook ham hock with water in covered soup kettle for 1 hour. Remove meat from bone and skin. Chop meat and put it back into water with the rest of the ingredients.

Simmer 40 minutes or more until soup is of desired consistency. (I simmer it several hours, until it becomes thick.) This freezes well. *Makes 8 cups.*

Nutrients per serving (without ham hock): Calories 60, Fat ½ g, Carbohydrate 12 g, Cholesterol 0, Sodium 220 mg, Fiber 3 g, Protein 4 g

Lentil Soup

Another hearty soup that freezes well. Since lentils contain vitamin E, which we miss in our avoidance of wheat, and also calcium, which many celiacs lose in avoidance of milk products, they are a good substitute.

2 cups lentils
2 quarts hot water
1 stalk celery, with leaves, chopped
1 medium onion, chopped
3 slices bacon, diced
1 clove garlic, minced
2 cloves
½ teaspoon oregano, crushed
Salt and pepper to taste

Cover lentils with hot water. There is no need to soak lentils. Add the celery, onion, bacon, garlic, cloves, and oregano to the lentils and place over high heat to bring to boil. Immediately reduce heat to a simmer and cook for 2½ to 3 hours, or until lentils are tender.

Remove the cloves. Add salt and pepper to taste (about 2 teaspoons salt and ⅛ teaspoon pepper) and serve or freeze. *Makes 6 to 8 servings.*

NOTE: To add flavor, substitute one 6-ounce can V8 juice for ¾ cup of the water.

Nutrients per serving: Calories 190, Fat 2 g, Carbohydrate 33 g, Cholesterol 15 mg, Sodium 170 mg, Fiber 4 g, Protein 11 g

Hillbilly Soup (16-Bean Soup)

This is an original Ozark recipe that calls for many kinds of beans. Don't worry if you can't find them all; any combination of some of these beans is fine. I buy the lot and then make up small plastic bags of 1½ cups each to cook later. Some I package with the recipe for gifts. Warning: *Some stores are selling these packages with barley as one of the ingredients.* Read the ingredient list.

Red kidney beans
Black-eyed peas
Garbanzo beans
Green split peas
Yellow split peas
Large navy beans
Baby limas
Small navy beans
Large white butter beans
Speckled limas
Field peas
Lentils
Pinto beans
Black beans
Pink beans
Small red beans

Wash 1½ cups bean mixture. Cover with water, add 1 tablespoon salt, and soak overnight. Drain.

Put soaked beans in 2 quarts water. (For added flavor, substitute one 6-ounce can V8 juice for ¾ cup water.) Add:

½ pound ham pieces
1 clove garlic, chopped
One 28-ounce can tomatoes
Juice of 1 lemon
Salt and pepper to taste
1 onion, chopped
1 green or red pepper, chopped (optional)

Bring to a simmer and let cook on low at least 4 hours. Check occasionally for liquid. As it cooks down it thickens. You can add water or not as you desire. I like the thicker soup and cook mine most of the day. The flavor improves with age. *Makes 8 to 10 servings.*

Nutrients per serving: Calories 630, Fat 6 g, Carbohydrate 105 g, Cholesterol 15 mg, Sodium 740 mg, Fiber 19 g, Protein 42 g

Where to Find Gluten-free Products

When I wrote *The Gluten-free Gourmet* a decade ago, the suppliers for products without gluten were very few, and the products they carried were limited. All that has changed, and today we can find over fifty large suppliers while more GF products are carried in health food stores and specialty markets. Many support groups sell the flours, mixes, and xanthan gum at their meetings or by mail order; otherwise you will find anything you need for baking from the list of suppliers below.

Even more exciting is the fact that in the last year or so, cake and bread mixes have joined the GF cookies and crackers on a few grocery shelves while Asian stores carry fine white rice, tapioca, and potato starch flours. And the mail-order suppliers have branched out into more than just cookies and mixes. Some furnish main dishes either frozen or freeze dried to eat at home or while camping; others provide ready-baked full desserts.

With these many suppliers specializing in gluten-free goods, you should find your baking needs close to home. But there are still a few flours featured in this new edition so unusual that they haven't reached regular markets (such as the Garfava and sorghum flours). They will have to be special ordered until the health food stores carry them on a regular basis.

Alpineaire Foods (freeze-dried soups, meals for camping, hiking, and backpacking): 4031 Alvis Court, Rocklin, CA 95677; (800) 322-6325 or

(916) 824-5000; fax (916) 824-5020. Accepts orders by mail, phone, and fax. Some products can be found in sporting goods stores. Write or phone for a full product list.

Authentic Foods (baking mixes for pancakes, bread, and cakes; Garfava flour, brown and white rice flour, tapioca starch, potato flour and potato starch, xanthan gum, maple sugar, vanilla powder, rye flavor powder): 1850 West 169th St., Suite B, Gardena, CA 90247; (800) 806-4737 or (310) 366-7612; fax (310) 366-6938. Accepts orders by phone, mail, and fax. Write for complete product list. Some products can be found in health food stores.

Bob's Red Mill Natural Foods (wheat-free biscuit and baking mix, xanthan and guar gum, wheat-free flours, legume flours): 5209 S. E. International Way, Milwaukie, OR 97222; (800) 553-2258; fax (503) 653-1339. Website *www.bobsredmill.com.* Takes orders by mail, phone, and fax. Write for an order form. Some products can be found in health food stores and in health sections of grocery stores.

Cybros, Inc. (white rice flour and tapioca flour): P.O. Box 851, Waukesha, WI 53187-0851; (800) 876-2253; fax (262) 547-8946. Accepts orders by mail or phone. Products can also be found in health food stores.

Dietary Specialties, Inc., a MenuDirect Company (crackers, baking mixes, prepared entrees, breads, snacks, pretzels, xanthan and guar gum, flavorings, dough enhancer): 865 Centennial Avenue, Piscataway, NJ 08854; (888) 636-MENU; website: *www.dietspec.com.* Accepts orders by phone and mail. Write or phone for list of products.

El Peto Products Ltd. (strictly gluten-free manufacturer and distributor of fresh-baked products, baking mixes, soups, pastas, gluten-free flours, cookbooks, snacks, and crackers; bean, rice, quinoa, millet, and other GF flours milled especially for them by The Mill Stone): 41 Shoemaker Street, Kitchener, Ontario N2E 3G9, Canada; (800) 387-4064;

fax (519) 748-5279; email *elpeto@golden.net*; website *www.elpeto.com.* Order by phone, fax, mail, or email. Some products can be found in specialty markets and health food stores.

Ener-G-Foods, Inc. (breads, rolls, buns, pizza shells, doughnuts, cookies, granola and bars; xanthan gum, methocel, dough enhancer, almond meal; tapioca, bean, rice, and other gluten-free flours, and Bette Hagman's flour mixes; Egg Replacer, Lacto-Free, and cookbooks): P.O. Box 84487, Seattle, WA 98124; (800) 331-5222; fax (206) 764-3398; website *www.ener-g.com.* Accepts orders by phone, mail, fax, and secure website. Phone for a catalog of their long list. Products can be found in some health food stores and specialty markets.

Food for Life Baking Company, Inc. (baked bread and muffins, pastas): P.O. Box 1434, Corona, CA 91718-1434; (800) 797-5090; fax (909) 279-1784. Accepts orders by mail. Write for their complete order form. Products can be found in the frozen food section of specialty and natural food stores under the Food for Life name.

The Food Merchants (polenta and polenta pastas): 7120 W. 117th Avenue, B-1, Broomfield, CO 80020; (303) 404-2691; fax (303) 469-9630. Accepts orders by mail. Some products can be found in health food stores and some groceries. Phone for full product list.

G Foods (cookies, breakfast bars, granola): 3536 17th Street, San Francisco, CA 94110; (415) 255-2139; fax (415) 863-3359. Accepts orders by mail, phone, and fax. Write or phone for the full order form.

The Gluten-Free Pantry, Inc. (gluten-free mixes, crackers, cookies, pastas, soups, and baking supplies such as xanthan gum, guar gum, dough enhancer, plus a long list of gluten-free flours including white, brown, and wild rice, garbanzo bean, and several corn flours): P.O. Box 840, Glastonbury, CT 06033; (800) 291-8386 or (860) 633-3826; fax (860) 633-6853; website *www.glutenfree.com.* Write or phone for their free catalog. Accepts orders by phone, mail, or fax.

GLUTINO.com (DE-RO-MA) (breads, bagels, pizzas, cookies, mixes, pastas, baked items, and gluten-free flours): 1118 Berlier, Laval, Quebec H7L 3R9, Canada; (450) 629-7689 or (800) 363-3438 (DIET); fax (450) 629-4781. Call, fax, or write for their full catalog. Many items can be found in health food and grocery stores. Also sold through celiac organizations. Website *www.glutino.com.*

Grain Process Enterprises, LTD. (Romano, navy, and garbanzo bean flour; yellow pea flour and other gluten-free flours including rice, buckwheat, millet, tapioca, potato, and arrowroot; xanthan and guar gums): 115 Commander Blvd., Scarborough, Ontario M1S 3M7, Canada; (416) 291-3226; fax (416) 291-2159. Write or phone for their list. Takes orders by mail, phone, and fax. Some products can be found in health food stores.

Jowar Foods (sorghum flour): P.O. Box 775, Vega, TX 79092; (806) 267-0820; fax (806) 267-0769. Accepts order by phone, mail, and fax. Sorghum flour can be found in some health food stores and specialty markets.

The King Arthur Flour Company, Inc. (rice and tapioca flours, potato starch, xanthan gum): P.O. Box 876, Norwich, VT 05055; (800) 827-6836; fax (800) 343-3002. Accpts orders by phone, fax, and mail. Request a free catalog.

Kinnikinnick Foods (breads, buns, bagels, doughnuts, cookies, pizza crusts, muffins, xanthan gum, guar gum; rice, corn, potato, bean, and soya flours; other baking supplies): 10306-112 Street, Edmonton, Alberta T5K 1N1, Canada; (877) 503-4466; fax (780) 421-0456; toll free 1-877-503-4466; email *info@kinnikinnick.com*; website *www.kinnikinnick.com*. Accepts orders by phone, mail, fax, and secure website. Offers home delivery of all products to most areas in North America. Some products may be found in health food stores and regular grocery stores in the alternative food section.

Mrs. Leeper's Pasta (gluten-free corn and rice pastas): 12455 Kerran Street, #200, Poway, CA 92064; (858) 486-1101; fax (858) 406-1770.

Sold through health food stores and some gourmet sections in large grocery stores under the label Mrs. Leeper's Pasta or Michelle's Natural. Write or phone to inquire about distributors in your area. Mail orders will be filled for those living too far from stores handling these products.

Legumes Plus, Inc. (lentil soups, chili, casserole and salad mixes): P.O. Box 383, Fairfield, WA 99012; (800) 845-1349; fax (509) 283-2314. Accepts orders by phone, mail, and fax. Some products can be found in health food and gourmet stores and specialty supermarkets.

Mendocino Gluten-Free Products, Inc. (bread mix, pancake and waffle mix, general purpose flour): P.O. Box 277, Willits, CA 95490-0277; (800) 297-5399; fax (707) 459-1834. Products marketed under Sylvan Border Farm label. Orders taken by phone, mail, and fax. Write or phone for a full order form. Some products may be found in health food and grocery stores.

Nancy's Natural Foods (long list of GF flours including sorghum and bean; xanthan gum, guar gum, milk powders and substitutes): 266 N.W. First Avenue, Suite A, Canby, OR 97013; (503) 266-3306; fax (503) 266-3306; email *nnfoods@juno.com*. Accepts orders by phone, mail, and email. Ask for their long list of GF baking supplies.

Pamela's Products, Inc. (cookies, biscotti, and baking mixes): 335 Allerton Avenue, South San Francisco, CA 94080; (650) 952-4546; fax (650) 742-6643. Accepts orders by mail. Many products will be found in natural food stores and some in grocery stores under "Pamela's" label. Write or phone for their full order form.

The Really Great Food Co. (rice and tapioca flours, xanthan gum): P.O. Box 319, Malverne, NY 11565; (800) 593-5377; fax (516) 593-9522. Accepts orders by mail, phone, and fax. Call or write for a full product list.

Red River Milling Company (formerly Sam Pierce Plant) (sorghum [milo], mung, and garbanzo [chickpea] flours): 801 Cumberland Street,

Vernon, TX 76384; (800) 419-9614 or (940) 553-1211; fax (940) 552-2772. Accepts orders by mail and phone. Products also sold through Miss Roben's (see below) and celiac organizations. Company mills only gluten-free products.

Miss Roben's (baking mixes, ready-to-eat products, cookbooks, pastas, a long line of GF flours including sorghum and GF mix, xanthan gum, guar gum, and other baking supplies plus free technical help and baking support): P.O. Box 1149, Frederick, MD 21702; (800) 891-0083; fax (301) 665-9584; email *missroben@msn.com*. Accepts orders by mail, phone, email, and fax.

Son's Milling (Romano bean flour and other GF flours): 6820 Kirkpatrick Crescent, Victoria, BC V8M 1Z8, Canada; (250) 544-1733; fax (604) 389-6719. Accepts orders by phone, mail, and fax. Write or call for complete list. Some products may be found in health food stores.

Specialty Food Shop (mixes, baked goods, pasta, crackers, soups, cookbooks, and a long line of gluten-free flours, xanthan gum, guar gum, rice, and corn bran): Radio Centre Plaza, Upper Level, 875 Main Street West, Hamilton, Ontario L8S 4P9, Canada; or 555 University Avenue, Toronto, Ontario, M5G 1X8; (800) SFS-7976 or (905) 528-4707 (Hamilton) or (416) 977-4360 (Toronto); fax (905) 528-5625 (Hamilton) or (416) 977-8394 (Toronto). Accepts orders by phone, mail, fax, and email (*www.specialtyfoodshop.com*). Write for product list. Also has retail stores in Hamilton and Toronto.

Sterk's Bakery (new French bread, dinner rolls, bagels, gluten-free flour, baking mixes, and more): 3866 23 Street, Jordan, Ontario, L0R 1S0, Canada, or 1402 Pine Avenue, Suite 727, Niagara Falls, NY, 14301; (905) 562-3086; fax (905) 562-3847. Accepts orders by mail and phone. Write for a free catalog.

Tad Enterprises (rice, potato, and tapioca flours, xanthan and guar gums, bread mix, cereal, pasta): 9356 Pleasant, Tinley Park, IL 60477;

(800) 438-6153; fax (708) 429-3954. Accepts orders by mail, phone, and fax. Write for order form for complete list of products.

Tamarind Tree (GF shelf stable, vegetarian, ready to heat and serve Indian entrees): 518 Justin Way, Neshanic Station, NJ 08853; (908) 369-6300; fax (908) 369-9300. Accepts orders by mail and phone. Products may be found in some health food stores. Check the website for list of products: *www.tamtree.com.*

This list, offered for the reader's convenience, was updated at the time of publication of this book. I regret I cannot be responsible for later changes in names, addresses, or phone numbers or for a company's removing some products from its line.

Index